Origin Stories

Supporting Identity Formation in Donor-Conceived
Children, Guiding parents, Educators, and Clinicians in
Helping Donor-conceived Children Build Strong, Integrated
Identities

Nicci Brochard
&
Dr. Ben Chuba

Origin Stories

Supporting Identity Formation in Donor-Conceived Children, Guiding parents, Educators, and Clinicians in Helping Donor-conceived Children Build Strong, Integrated Identities

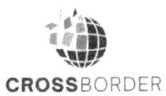

CROSSBORDER

New York, London, Quebec

Contents

Introduction

In an era of rapid advancements in reproductive technology, the concept of donor conception has become increasingly common. Donor-conceived children, who are brought into the world through sperm, egg, or embryo donation, represent a growing segment of society. While the medical, legal, and ethical implications of donor conception are often discussed, one area that requires more attention is the psychological and emotional development of these children, particularly when it comes to identity formation. "Origin Stories: Supporting Identity Formation in Donor-Conceived Children" seeks to address this gap by offering guidance to parents, educators, and clinicians on how to help donor-conceived children build strong, integrated identities that honor both their biological and social connections.

Identity formation is one of the most important developmental tasks in childhood. For all children, the process of understanding who they are involves navigating a complex web of relationships, personal traits, family history, and cultural influences. For donor-conceived children, however, there are additional layers of complexity, as these children may not have direct knowledge of one or both of their biological parents. This absence of a direct connection to their genetic origins can lead to questions of belonging, self-worth, and a sense of wholeness. Children may struggle to reconcile the love and care they receive from their social parents with the curiosity and sometimes longing for information about their biological roots.

The task of supporting a donor-conceived child's identity development requires a nuanced understanding of their unique needs. This book is designed to provide a comprehensive framework for parents, educators, and clinicians, offering them the tools to foster a healthy and integrated sense of self in these children. It recognizes that identity formation is not a one-time event but an ongoing process that continues to evolve throughout a child's life. Thus, the support systems in place for these children must be flexible, responsive, and open to the child's developmental stages.

One of the key themes explored in this book is the importance of open and honest communication. Research has shown that children who are aware of their donor conception from an early age and have access to age-appropriate information are better able to navigate the complexities of their identity. Keeping the lines of communication open allows for the child to explore their feelings about their origins without fear of judgment or rejection. Parents and caregivers are encouraged to adopt an open and accepting approach when discussing the subject of donor conception. They should be prepared to offer support, answer questions, and, when necessary, seek out professional guidance to help them address sensitive topics with care.

The book also explores the emotional challenges that donor-conceived children may face as they grow older, particularly as they begin to understand the implications of their origins in relation to broader social and cultural contexts. Many donor-conceived children experience a sense of "otherness" when they encounter individuals who share a genetic connection to them, whether through DNA testing or through meeting biological relatives. Educators and clinicians need to be aware of these challenges and equipped to provide a supportive and non-judgmental space for children to process their emotions.

Importantly, "Origin Stories" emphasizes the role of community in supporting a donor-conceived child's identity development. Families, schools, and healthcare providers must work together to create environments where these children feel accepted and understood. A collaborative approach ensures that donor-conceived children are not only supported in their quest for self-knowledge but are also surrounded by a network of individuals who respect and affirm their personal journeys.

"Origin Stories: Supporting Identity Formation in Donor-Conceived Children" provides invaluable insights for anyone involved in the life of a donor-conceived child. Through thoughtful guidance and practical strategies, this book empowers parents, educators, and clinicians to help these children build resilient and integrated identities that honor both their donor conception and the families who raise them. By embracing the complexity of identity formation in the context of donor conception, we can ensure that these children grow up with a strong sense of self, connection, and belonging.

Nicci and I (Ben) thank you immensely for choosing our book. We promise you will find it helpful and supportive.

Chapter 1

What Makes Us Who We Are?

Introduction:

The question of "What makes us who we are?" has intrigued philosophers, psychologists, biologists, and even everyday people for centuries. From a scientific standpoint, it's the intersection of multiple factors—our genes, the environment we grow up in, the stories we tell about ourselves, and the relationships we form—that come together to shape the complexity of human identity. At the core of this exploration is the realization that no single aspect of our existence can fully explain who we become. Identity is not a static trait that we inherit or develop through a single path. Instead, it's a dynamic, multifaceted process shaped by a multitude of forces and experiences.

For donor-conceived children, the puzzle of identity can be even more complex. These children are born of genetic material donated by individuals who may not have an active role in their lives. In these cases, the typical narrative of family and biological inheritance becomes intertwined with questions of belonging, legacy, and self-discovery. As society continues to evolve in its understanding of genetics and reproductive technologies, the unique path of donor-conceived children requires careful attention. This chapter takes a deep dive into the multifaceted forces that shape identity, starting with the foundation of identity itself and moving towards the unique experiences of donor-conceived children. We will explore how the forces of nature and nurture interact, how identity is constructed through storytelling, and why understanding the unique journey of donor-conceived children matters for both them and the people who support them.

Section 1: The Foundations of Identity

Genes, Environment, and Storytelling

Identity is a blend of our genetic makeup, the environments we are raised in, and the stories we craft about ourselves. Let's break down these three primary components.

Genetics: From the moment we are conceived, our genetic code begins to lay the groundwork for who we will become. Our genes influence everything from the color of our eyes to our risk of developing certain diseases, and they can even have subtle impacts on our personality traits. We are, in many ways, a product of the genes passed down to us from our biological parents. This biological inheritance is often regarded as the "nature" part of the identity equation.

However, genes do not solely define us. While genetic predispositions may offer a general blueprint for development, they are not destiny. The environment into which we are born plays an equally important role in shaping who we become. This brings us to the second element: environment.

Environment: The environment we grow up in—our family dynamics, culture, socioeconomic status, education, and social relationships—exerts profound influence on our development. The way we are nurtured impacts our behavior, choices, emotional health, and even how we relate to our genetic inheritance. For example, a child born into a supportive and loving environment is likely to develop a different sense of self than one raised in an environment filled with neglect or emotional distress. It is through this interaction with the world around us that we begin to make sense of ourselves, our relationships, and our place in the world.

Storytelling: Lastly, identity is shaped by the stories we tell. These narratives are often constructed in relation to the people around us and the experiences we accumulate over time. From a young age, we begin to weave stories about who we are—our family history, our cultural identity, our triumphs and challenges. We also inherit stories from others. Families tell stories of ancestors and traditions, often framing our identity in a cultural context. For donor-conceived children, the stories told by their families may focus on how they came into the world, the role of the donor, and how this information is integrated into the larger narrative of who they are.

It is through these stories that we come to understand ourselves and our place in the world. For donor-conceived children, the narrative becomes especially important as they attempt to reconcile their biological origins with their social and familial identity. In the next section, we will explore how these foundational elements of identity—genes, environment, and storytelling—interact in the context of donor conception.

Section 2: The Unique Path of Donor-Conceived Children

Origins with a Twist: Conceived but Not Forgotten

For donor-conceived children, the traditional models of identity formation face unique challenges. These children inherit their genetic material from one or more donors who are often unknown to them, leading to a distinction between their genetic and social heritage. The significance of this distinction cannot be overstated.

Unlike children born through traditional means, where a direct connection to both biological parents is immediately understood, donor-conceived children face the reality that one biological parent—the donor—is absent. For many of these children, the donor's absence can evoke feelings of confusion, loss, and a longing to understand their origins. The donor-conceived child is left to reconcile the genetic piece of their identity with the story of their upbringing, as told by their social parents.

While genetics undoubtedly play a significant role in shaping the child's physical traits, intelligence, and temperament, the absence of one biological parent often leaves a psychological void. Questions about their donor's identity—whether or not they share any personality traits or health conditions, or whether they might have a deeper, emotional connection—are not easily answered. This absence of information can create challenges in the formation of a cohesive identity, as the child may feel incomplete without access to their full biological background.

This dynamic makes the process of identity formation for donor-conceived children particularly intriguing. Their sense of self doesn't fit neatly into the traditional narrative of inheritance, where identity is derived from a concrete family structure. Instead, their identity is often a patchwork of known and unknown factors, shaped by their social family environment and the information they can piece together about their biological heritage.

Why Their Story Matters

The stories of donor-conceived children matter because they illuminate the complexities of human identity and the profound impact that both genetic and social factors have on development. When it comes to understanding donor-conceived children, it's critical to shift our perspective from a purely genetic viewpoint to one that considers the emotional and psychological implications of their unique origins.

For parents, educators, and clinicians, understanding the complexities of donor conception is crucial to supporting these children in their journey of self-discovery. Many donor-conceived children begin their lives without knowledge of their genetic origins, and some may even grow up feeling disconnected from the donor's family history. The process of uncovering this unknown story—whether through genetic testing, finding a donor sibling, or gaining access to additional family medical history—can be an emotionally charged and sometimes confusing process.

The importance of offering a supportive environment for donor-conceived children to explore their origins cannot be overstated. It is critical for families to understand that identity formation in these children is a multifaceted, ongoing process. While genetic heritage is important, it is the context in which a child is raised, the stories that are told, and the emotional connections they form that truly shape who they are.

Providing donor-conceived children with a sense of control over their own narrative is equally important. This means creating opportunities for open discussions about their origins, ensuring that they have access to information when they are ready, and allowing them to ask questions without fear of rejection or invalidation. In doing so, we can help these children develop a positive and integrated sense of identity, one that acknowledges both their biological and social heritage.

Conclusion

The exploration of what makes us who we are takes us into the heart of identity formation—an intricate dance between genetics, environment, and the stories we tell about ourselves. For donor-conceived children, this process is further complicated by the absence of one biological parent and the presence of unknowns that can impact their understanding of self. As we've seen, the intersection of genetic material, nurturing environments, and personal storytelling plays a central role in shaping a child's identity, especially for those with a unique conception story.

Supporting donor-conceived children in their identity formation is an ongoing, dynamic process that requires sensitivity, empathy, and understanding. By acknowledging the complexities of their experiences and providing a foundation of open communication and supportive relationships, we can help these children form strong, integrated identities that honor both their biological and social roots. Ultimately, the story of donor-conceived children is not just about genetics or family history—it's about the resilience of human identity, the power of personal narratives, and the importance of belonging in all its forms.

Chapter 2

The Donor Conception Landscape

Introduction:

The world of donor conception is a complex one, shaped by a combination of medical advancements, legal frameworks, societal attitudes, and ethical considerations. For many donor-conceived children, understanding their origins requires not only a deep exploration of their personal stories but also an awareness of the broader historical and global context in which their conception took place. This chapter seeks to provide a comprehensive overview of the donor conception landscape, starting with its historical evolution, followed by a discussion of the global perspectives on donor conception.

In the first section, we will explore the evolution of donor conception, beginning with its secretive and often hidden beginnings, and moving through to the more open dialogues of today. We will delve into the rise of reproductive technologies, examining how advances in assisted reproductive technologies (ART) have transformed the way families are made. In the second section, we will broaden the discussion to the global picture, where donor conception is viewed through different lenses across cultures, laws, and regulations. This section will also look at the differing approaches to anonymous and open donation across countries, and how these practices reflect cultural values surrounding family, genetics, and identity.

Section 1: A Brief History

From Secretive Beginnings to Open Dialogues

The history of donor conception is far more secretive than most people realize. In the early years of artificial insemination (AI) and sperm donation, the practice was carried out in an atmosphere of confidentiality, secrecy, and even shame. This secrecy was rooted in social taboos about infertility, the role of women in reproduction, and the sanctity of traditional family structures. Sperm donation, in particular, was often seen as a last resort for couples who had failed to conceive naturally, and there was little to no discussion about the identity of the donor or the implications for the child born from such a union.

As early as the 1940s and 1950s, doctors began experimenting with artificial insemination using donor sperm, but these procedures were often done in private settings, and donors were kept anonymous. The assumption was that the child would never learn about their donor parentage, and the couple using the donor sperm would raise the child as their own. The child's genetics were considered irrelevant to their sense of identity, and the social parents were thought to be the only "true" parents. The psychological impact of growing up without knowledge of one's genetic origins was rarely considered, and parents were advised to keep the donor conception secret, creating a hidden layer of their family's history.

This period of secrecy began to shift in the 1970s and 1980s, as the medical community, along with growing advocacy from reproductive rights groups, started to push for a more open dialogue about assisted reproduction. As fertility treatments such as in vitro fertilization (IVF) became more widespread, there was a growing recognition that transparency was necessary. Children born through donor conception were increasingly seen as having the right to know their genetic origins, and many parents began to reconsider the idea of secrecy. This change was also driven by the recognition of the potential psychological harm of keeping such an important part of a child's identity hidden from them.

With the advent of the internet in the 1990s and 2000s, the issue of donor conception became more public, and families started to share their stories. Websites and online forums allowed donor-conceived individuals to connect, share their experiences, and even search for biological relatives. These changes sparked a broader cultural conversation about the ethics of donor conception, the rights of children to know their origins, and the implications of genetic heritage. As a result, many countries began to reconsider their approach to donor anonymity.

The Rise of Reproductive Technologies

Reproductive technologies have revolutionized the landscape of donor conception, offering new possibilities for individuals and couples struggling with infertility. The first successful in vitro fertilization (IVF) birth in 1978 marked the beginning of a new era in assisted reproductive technologies. IVF, along with other treatments like intrauterine insemination (IUI), egg donation, and embryo donation, provided families with options that were previously unavailable.

These advances not only allowed more people to have children, but they also introduced a broader range of family-building possibilities. IVF and sperm donation, for example, opened doors for single women, same-sex couples, and heterosexual couples facing male infertility to have biological children. As reproductive technologies continued to develop, the need for a larger pool of donors also increased, which led to the creation of sperm banks and egg banks that could provide anonymous donors to individuals in need.

As ART has become more mainstream, its societal and legal implications have also come into focus. The growing use of ART has brought questions of donor anonymity, parental rights, the regulation of sperm banks, and the protection of donor-conceived children's rights to the forefront. While some countries continue to maintain anonymous donation policies, others have moved toward open donation, where donors are known to the children they help create, and children have access to donor information when they reach a certain age. The rise of reproductive technologies has led to a shift from secrecy toward transparency, and from a focus on the interests of parents to a greater emphasis on the rights of the child.

Section 2: The Global Picture

Regulations, Laws, and Cultural Differences

Donor conception is not a universal practice, and the laws governing it vary significantly across countries. Different cultural values, ethical beliefs, and legal frameworks shape how donor conception is perceived and practiced worldwide. In some countries, donor conception is tightly regulated, with strict laws about donor anonymity, while in others, it is more loosely regulated, with fewer restrictions on the identity of the donor or the rights of the child.

For example, in the United States, sperm donation is primarily regulated at the state level, with some states requiring donor screening and others offering less oversight. The U.S. has a largely unregulated market for sperm and egg donation, leading to widespread anonymity in many cases. However, in countries like the United Kingdom, Sweden, and Australia, donor conception is much more heavily regulated, and there are laws that allow children born through donor conception to access identifying information about their donors once they reach adulthood. These policies reflect a broader cultural shift towards prioritizing the rights of the child over the rights of the parents or the donors.

In many European countries, including the Netherlands and Norway, anonymous sperm donation is prohibited, and donors are required to provide identifying information that can be shared with children born from their donations. These regulations reflect a cultural belief in the importance of children knowing their genetic origins and having the right to access that information. In contrast, countries like Japan and some parts of the Middle East have more conservative views on donor conception and may impose greater restrictions on the practice, sometimes limiting the use of donor sperm or egg for unmarried individuals or same-sex couples.

Anonymous vs. Open Donation Across Countries

The practice of anonymous versus open donation is a significant point of divergence in global attitudes toward donor conception. Some countries continue to permit anonymous donation, where the donor's identity is kept confidential, and the children conceived through the donation have no legal or moral claim to any information about their biological parent. This practice was once the standard in many parts of the world, but it has been increasingly challenged by advocates for the rights of donor-conceived individuals, who argue that every child has the right to know their biological heritage.

In countries like the UK, Sweden, and New Zealand, open donation is now the norm. In these countries, donors are required to provide identifying information, and children conceived through their donations have the right to contact them once they reach adulthood. The idea behind open donation is that it allows for greater transparency and gives the donor-conceived child access to information that is critical for understanding their biological origins and family medical history.

However, there are still many countries where anonymous donation is the preferred model. In some cases, this is due to cultural or religious beliefs that prioritize family privacy and the traditional family unit. In these countries, the focus remains on the social family—the parents who raise the child—rather than the genetic origins of the child. The idea of a child having access to identifying information about a donor may be seen as unnecessary or even disruptive to family cohesion.

The Global Debate: Balancing Rights and Ethics

The global landscape of donor conception is marked by a constant tension between ethical considerations, legal frameworks, and the evolving rights of donor-conceived children. The debate between anonymous and open donation continues to stir strong emotions, with supporters of each model citing valid concerns. Proponents of anonymous donation argue that it respects the privacy of donors and allows for the continued availability of sperm and egg donations without complex legal or emotional entanglements. Those in favor of open donation emphasize the rights of donor-conceived children to know their biological origins, arguing that access to donor information is crucial for the child's identity formation, health considerations, and understanding of their family history.

Ultimately, the global picture of donor conception remains in flux, with different countries finding their own balance between medical practice, legal frameworks, and cultural values. As the world continues to grapple with these issues, it's clear that the landscape of donor conception will continue to evolve, influenced by changing societal norms, advances in reproductive technology, and an ever-deepening understanding of the psychological and emotional needs of donor-conceived children.

Conclusion

The journey of donor conception, from its secretive beginnings to the increasingly open and regulated practices we see today, highlights both the complexities and the progress that have been made in this field. Advances in reproductive technologies have allowed for broader access to donor conception, but they have also sparked significant debates about anonymity, identity, and the rights of donor-conceived children. Across the globe, the regulation and practice of donor conception vary, influenced by cultural attitudes, ethical beliefs, and legal structures. As society continues to evolve, so too will the frameworks that govern donor conception, ensuring that the voices of donor-conceived children are heard and their rights respected in the ongoing conversation about family, identity, and genetics.

Chapter 3

The Psychology of Knowing and Not Knowing

Introduction:

The question of biological ties holds immense psychological significance in the development of a child's identity. For most children, their understanding of who they are begins with the knowledge of their biological parents. These parents are the individuals with whom they share their first physical and emotional connections. However, for donor-conceived children, the situation is often much more complex. Their biological ties may not align with their social parents, and in many cases, they may not even have access to the identity of their biological parent. The psychology of knowing and not knowing one's biological origins presents unique challenges and opportunities for self-understanding, attachment, and identity formation.

In this chapter, we explore the intricate psychological landscape that donor-conceived children navigate in relation to their biological ties. Section 1 delves into the role of these biological connections—how they shape attachment, influence identity formation, and can contribute to feelings of difference or incompleteness when unknown. Section 2 examines the silent struggle that many donor-conceived children experience, particularly the emotional confusion and curiosity that arise from not knowing the identity of one's biological parent. Through case studies, we will explore how these feelings manifest in real-life experiences and how they affect the child's sense of self.

Section 1: The Role of Biological Ties

Attachment, Identity, and Genetic Connection

Attachment theory, first developed by John Bowlby, emphasizes the deep emotional bonds that form between children and their caregivers. These bonds, rooted in the early years of life, play a fundamental role in shaping a child's emotional security, sense of self, and ability to form healthy relationships later in life. The attachment between a child and their parents is seen as one of the most important factors in the development of a stable and integrated identity. This emotional connection serves as the foundation upon which a child builds their sense of belonging, love, and worth.

However, when it comes to donor-conceived children, there is an additional layer to this attachment process. For many donor-conceived children, the relationship with their social parents remains the primary emotional bond, while the relationship with their biological parent is either unknown or distant. The question then arises: what role does the genetic connection to a biological parent play in shaping the child's identity?

Research on identity development consistently suggests that knowledge of biological roots can have a significant impact on an individual's sense of self. Biological ties, in particular, serve as a key component of identity because they anchor a person's sense of belonging to a specific family, culture, and history. For donor-conceived children, however, this genetic link is often either unknown or intentionally concealed. The absence of access to this information can lead to a sense of fragmentation, as the child may not be able to fully integrate their biological origins into their understanding of who they are.

Attachment to social parents is, of course, an essential factor in shaping the emotional and social development of donor-conceived children. These children often grow up in loving homes where they are fully integrated into family life, with their social parents serving as their primary caregivers. However, without the knowledge of their biological parent, the child may feel like an incomplete puzzle piece. This sense of incompleteness may stem from a subtle feeling that they are missing a part of their identity—something that connects them to a broader genetic or familial history.

In the absence of this knowledge, donor-conceived children may feel an innate longing or curiosity about their genetic origins, which can lead to questions about their place in the world. This feeling of "missing something" can manifest in various ways, such as a vague sense of not quite fitting in, or feeling different from family members or peers in ways that are hard to articulate. These feelings can sometimes be exacerbated when the child begins to develop a more acute awareness of their genetic origins, particularly during adolescence when the quest for self-understanding intensifies.

Feeling "Different" Without Knowing Why

For many donor-conceived children, the sensation of feeling "different" can be a constant, underlying experience. Without knowing their biological origins, these children may struggle to explain the sense of disconnection they feel, especially as they grow older and begin to compare themselves to others. This feeling of difference can be compounded by the realization that they do not have access to the same familial history that other children may have. For example, many children can trace their family lineage, medical history, and cultural background back for generations. They know the stories of their grandparents, great-grandparents, and extended family, and these stories become part of the fabric of their identity. Donor-conceived children, on the other hand, may feel left out of this shared narrative.

Adolescence is a particularly critical period for donor-conceived children when these feelings of difference may become more pronounced. During this developmental stage, children often begin to examine who they are in relation to their peers and family. They may notice physical characteristics, mannerisms, or even personality traits that don't seem to align with those of their social parents. These differences may provoke questions about their biological origins, which can lead to feelings of confusion, curiosity, or even frustration. The absence of an immediate, straightforward answer can create a sense of internal conflict for the child, who may not know where to turn for clarity.

The lack of knowledge about one's biological parent can also manifest as an unspoken and unacknowledged gap in the child's life story.

This silent struggle is often not addressed directly, as parents may be reluctant to bring up the topic of donor conception, fearing it will upset the child or disrupt the family dynamic. This silence can create an emotional barrier, leaving the child with a sense of alienation and a lack of control over their own narrative.

Section 2: The Silent Struggle

Confusion, Curiosity, and the Invisible Gap

The psychological impact of not knowing one's biological origins can be profound. While social parents provide love, care, and support, the child may still experience a sense of absence—a gap in their story that they are unable to fill. This silent struggle can lead to confusion, as the child grapples with the question of who they truly are. They may wonder why they feel disconnected from their family history, or why certain aspects of their personality don't seem to align with the people they call family.

Curiosity often accompanies this confusion. The desire to know more about one's biological parent(s) is a natural and deeply human need. This curiosity may start as an innocent question about physical traits or family health history, but it can quickly evolve into a more profound longing to understand the roots of one's identity. For many donor-conceived children, this curiosity intensifies over time, especially as they reach adulthood. Some may turn to genetic testing or online databases in an attempt to uncover the identity of their biological parent, while others may seek out donor siblings or engage in social media communities for donor-conceived individuals.

Unfortunately, this quest for information can be complicated by the legal and ethical frameworks that govern donor conception. In many cases, donors are anonymized, and children are prohibited from accessing identifying information. These legal restrictions can heighten feelings of frustration and helplessness, as the child is left to navigate the complexities of their identity without the necessary resources or support.

Case Studies: Children Who Felt the Disconnect

The emotional challenges faced by donor-conceived children are well-documented in case studies. One case involved a young woman named Sarah, who had always known she was donor-conceived, but it wasn't until she entered her teenage years that she began to feel a sense of disconnection from her social parents. Sarah began to notice physical traits in herself—such as her height and eye color—that were different from those of her family members. Despite being loved and nurtured by her parents, she began to feel like something was missing, like she was somehow "other."

Sarah's curiosity grew as she questioned the absence of her biological father. She wanted to know where her genetic traits came from, but her parents were hesitant to provide answers. They had always kept her donor conception a secret, and now, they were unsure how to approach the topic. Sarah's emotional distress deepened as she felt she could not truly understand herself without this missing piece of information. Eventually, Sarah took matters into her own hands and found a way to access her donor's identity, which brought both relief and new emotional challenges. Although she was grateful to know more about her biological origins, she struggled with the implications of this new knowledge and the emotional complexity it brought into her family life.

Another case study involved David, a young man who had no idea he was donor-conceived until he was in his twenties. David had always been told that he was adopted, but the details of his adoption were unclear. When he eventually discovered that he was conceived through sperm donation, he felt betrayed by his parents for keeping this secret. His feelings of confusion turned into anger as he tried to reconcile his family identity with the reality of his biological origins. David's journey of self-discovery was complicated by his emotions about his biological father, whom he could never know. The emotional struggle of navigating this new chapter in his life was intense, and it took years of therapy for him to integrate this knowledge into his broader sense of self.

Conclusion

The psychology of knowing and not knowing one's biological ties is a deeply complex and emotional journey for donor-conceived children. Attachment to social parents is a critical component of their identity development, but the absence of knowledge about their biological parent can create feelings of fragmentation and confusion. As we have seen through the case studies, these children often experience a silent struggle—a gap in their story that leads to curiosity, longing, and, in some cases, frustration. It is essential to provide support and open communication for donor-conceived children, helping them navigate their unique psychological challenges and facilitating a healthy integration of their biological and social identities. Understanding the psychology of knowing and not knowing is the first step in ensuring that donor-conceived children are given the tools to build strong, integrated identities that honor both their social and biological origins.

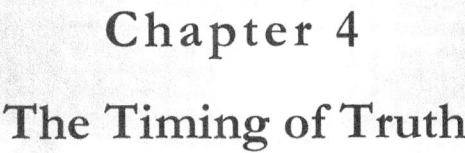

Chapter 4

The Timing of Truth

Introduction:

The decision of when and how to tell a child they are donor-conceived is one of the most profound challenges parents can face. It is a question that brings with it deep emotional significance, touching upon issues of identity, family dynamics, and the intricate process of truth-telling itself. This revelation can shape the way a child views their place in the world and their relationship with their family. When delivered in the right way, the truth can become a powerful tool for self-understanding and empowerment. When mishandled, however, it can sow confusion, insecurity, and a sense of betrayal.

In the world of donor conception, there are no one-size-fits-all solutions. The timing of such a discussion is influenced by many factors, including the child's age, their cognitive and emotional development, the family's cultural values, and the parents' own comfort levels with the subject. This chapter will explore the nuances of when and how to have this important conversation, addressing the ongoing debate between early disclosure and delayed conversations, the role of a child's cognitive development in determining the best time to talk, and the tools parents can use to make the conversation as safe, open, and positive as possible.

As parents, educators, and clinicians, understanding the complexities of timing and communication can lead to more supportive, thoughtful, and empathetic approaches to donor-conceived children's experiences. This chapter will guide you through the psychological and emotional layers of disclosure and offer strategies for ensuring that the truth is delivered with care, compassion, and clarity.

Section 1: When to Tell

Early Disclosure vs. Delayed Conversations

The question of whether to tell a child early in life or wait until they are older is a dilemma that many parents of donor-conceived children face. Both approaches have their merits, and the decision often depends on a range of personal and practical factors.

Early Disclosure: The primary advantage of early disclosure is that it allows for transparency from the start, preventing the child from ever feeling that there is a "secret" about their conception. By introducing the concept of donor conception at a young age, parents set the tone for openness and honesty. This approach also ensures that the child's identity development is not disrupted later on by a surprise revelation.

From a psychological perspective, children as young as three or four can begin to understand simple concepts about family and genetics. Early disclosure, when done appropriately, can help normalize the child's experience. For example, parents might say things like, "You were born with help from a very special person who wanted to help create you," or "You were made with love by your donor and by us." By using age-appropriate language, these early conversations can frame donor conception as just another way that families are made.

The key benefit of early disclosure is that the child grows up with a clear sense of their origins. There is no hidden knowledge that might later be perceived as a betrayal. The child has the time to absorb the information in small, manageable doses and can ask questions when they are ready. This approach can also help prevent feelings of confusion or mistrust that might arise if the child learns about their donor conception in their teenage years or later, which is often when identity and self-concept are being more solidly formed.

However, early disclosure does require parents to engage with the topic from the outset, which can feel daunting, especially when the parents themselves may not have fully processed their own feelings about donor conception. It may feel unnatural for some parents to speak openly about such an intimate topic. Moreover, early disclosure requires ongoing conversations as the child matures, adjusting the language and content to fit their growing understanding.

Delayed Conversations: On the other hand, some parents opt to delay the conversation until the child is older, believing that the child will better understand the complexity of the situation once they are capable of grasping abstract concepts such as genetics, biological relationships, and family structure. For example, by the age of seven or eight, many children have developed a more sophisticated understanding of biology and family dynamics. At this stage, parents may feel that the child is more capable of understanding the nuances of donor conception, including the role of a donor in the child's biological makeup.

This approach may be particularly appealing to parents who want to avoid overwhelming their child with information before they are developmentally ready. Waiting until the child is older allows parents to gauge the child's emotional readiness and ensures that the information can be conveyed in a way that is more likely to be understood and processed.

However, the challenge with delayed disclosure is the potential for the child to experience feelings of betrayal or confusion later on. If the child discovers the truth on their own or hears it from someone else, the revelation may feel like a secret that has been kept from them for too long. This can lead to a sense of disillusionment or hurt, especially during adolescence, when issues of identity are particularly salient. Adolescence is a time of self-discovery and exploration of familial bonds, and for many donor-conceived children, learning that they are donor-conceived at this stage can be a shock to their sense of self.

Another consideration in delayed disclosure is that the longer the topic remains unspoken, the more difficult it may become for parents to broach it. It may feel awkward or uncomfortable to introduce the subject, particularly if the child has already reached an age where they might have questions about their origins. This may be compounded by guilt or shame that the parents feel about not having been open from the beginning.

The Child's Age and Cognitive Development

One of the most important factors to consider when deciding when to tell a child about their donor conception is the child's age and cognitive development. The ability to understand complex concepts such as genetics, family structure, and biological versus social relationships varies with age. Therefore, parents must consider the developmental stage of their child when deciding how to introduce the subject.

Young Children (3-5 years): At this stage, children's understanding of family and relationships is concrete and often based on the people who are immediately present in their lives. Their cognitive abilities are still developing, so the concept of donor conception may not make sense to them right away. However, young children can begin to understand simple facts, such as "You were made with the help of a donor," or "Your donor is part of your story." Conversations at this age should focus on basic, positive information, using simple language and gentle explanations. This early introduction sets the groundwork for later, more complex discussions as the child matures.

Elementary School Children (6-12 years): By this stage, children are capable of understanding more abstract concepts, including biological relationships and differences in family structures. They can begin to grasp the difference between biological and social parents and may start to ask more questions about where they came from and why they look or act differently from other family members. Conversations at this age should be more detailed, and parents should be prepared to explain the role of the donor in the child's life. While the child's understanding will continue to evolve, this is a good time to introduce the topic in a straightforward manner.

Adolescents (13+ years): Adolescence is a time when identity formation becomes especially crucial. Adolescents are capable of understanding the full complexity of donor conception, including the emotional, psychological, and social aspects of their origins. However, by this age, if the child has not been informed previously, the conversation may come as a shock. The child may feel betrayed or confused, especially if they have developed a strong sense of self based on other narratives about their family. Conversations with adolescents should be open, honest, and empathetic. Parents should be prepared for a range of emotional responses, from curiosity and acceptance to anger or sadness. The key is to create an environment where the adolescent feels comfortable expressing their emotions and asking questions.

In addition to age, parents should also consider the cognitive development of the child. Some children mature earlier than others, and some may be more ready to handle difficult topics at a younger age. Parents should be attuned to their child's emotional cues and readiness for such conversations, regardless of age.

Section 2: How to Tell

Scripts, Storybooks, and Safe Language

Once parents have decided when to have the conversation, the next important consideration is how to tell the child. The way in which the truth is communicated can deeply impact the child's emotional response and their sense of self. It is essential to choose language that is age-appropriate, non-judgmental, and reassuring.

One powerful tool in this regard is scripts—carefully constructed phrases or narratives that can help parents navigate the conversation with clarity and sensitivity. These scripts should focus on the positives of donor conception, emphasizing that the child is loved and wanted. For example, a script for younger children might be: "You were born with the help of a special person who gave us a gift so that we could become a family. That person helped create you, but you are our child, and we love you so much."

As children grow older, the language can become more complex, but it should always be framed in a positive, affirming way. For older children, a script might sound like: "You were conceived with the help of a donor, someone who gave us the gift of life so that we could have you. We love you exactly as you are, and your donor is just one part of your story. You are our child, and nothing will ever change that."

In addition to using scripts, storybooks are another effective tool for conveying the message of donor conception in a way that is accessible and comforting to children. Storybooks often present the information in a neutral, non-threatening way, using fictional characters to explain donor conception in an age-appropriate manner. These books often include reassuring messages about the child's place in the family, reinforcing the idea that the child's value is not determined by biology but by the love and care they receive from their family.

Finally, it is essential to use safe language throughout the conversation. This means avoiding any words or phrases that might make the child feel ashamed or less-than. The narrative should always emphasize that the child's identity is valid, whole, and deeply loved, regardless of how they came into the world. Avoiding shame and guilt is crucial in helping the child form a healthy, integrated sense of self.

Avoiding Shame and Guilt in the Narrative

The most important aspect of telling a child about their donor conception is ensuring that the conversation is framed in a way that avoids introducing any feelings of shame or guilt. Children must not feel as though their existence is a burden or a mistake. They need to understand that they are loved unconditionally, and their biological origins do not define their worth.

To avoid these negative emotions, parents should be mindful of the tone and content of the conversation. Phrases that might imply the child is somehow "different" or "less than" due to their conception should be avoided at all costs. The focus should always remain on the child's value as a person and their importance to the family.

In addition, parents should be prepared to address any feelings of shame or guilt that may arise in the child. This may require multiple conversations over time, allowing the child to express their feelings and ask questions. By consistently affirming the child's worth and reinforcing their place in the family, parents can help their child develop a strong, positive sense of self.

Conclusion

The timing and approach to telling a child about their donor conception are crucial factors in how the child processes this information and incorporates it into their identity. Early disclosure can provide a sense of transparency and prevent confusion later on, while delayed conversations may be more appropriate for some children based on their cognitive and emotional readiness. Regardless of the timing, it is essential that the conversation be framed in a positive, affirming manner, using age-appropriate language and tools such as scripts, storybooks, and safe language.

By creating an environment that is open, supportive, and free from shame, parents can ensure that their donor-conceived children feel valued, loved, and secure in their identity. The truth about donor conception, when shared with care and compassion, can become a powerful tool for self-understanding and acceptance, empowering the child to embrace their full story and integrate all aspects of their identity with pride.

Chapter 5

Identity in the Age of DNA Tests

Introduction:

The rapid advancement of genetic testing has changed the way we view identity, family, and heritage. Services like 23andMe, Ancestry.com, and other DNA testing platforms have made it easier than ever to discover one's genetic background, connect with distant relatives, and, in some cases, uncover family secrets. For many, these tests have become a fascinating tool for self-discovery, offering a deeper understanding of one's origins. However, for donor-conceived individuals, these DNA tests represent a new frontier in identity formation—one that can lead to unexpected and sometimes startling revelations.

This chapter explores the impact of genetic testing on identity, particularly for children who may learn new truths about their biological origins through DNA testing. In Section 1, we will examine the new normal of discovery, exploring how DNA testing services have made it easier for people to find out more about their biological connections, sometimes leading to unexpected truths. This section will also look at stories of sudden reveals and reunions, illustrating the emotional and psychological effects of these discoveries. In Section 2, we will focus on how to empower children who discover unexpected roots, offering guidance on how to support them in processing these revelations and how to navigate the legal, emotional, and practical steps that may follow. In a world where the truth about one's origins can be just a DNA test away, understanding how to approach these discoveries with care and support is crucial for healthy identity development.

Section 1: The New Normal of Discovery

23andMe, Ancestry, and Accidental Truths

The rise of commercial genetic testing companies like 23andMe, Ancestry.com, and MyHeritage has transformed the way we think about family and ancestry. What was once a subject reserved for genealogical enthusiasts or those with specific family histories has now become an activity accessible to anyone with an internet connection and a desire to learn more about their roots. These platforms have empowered people to trace their family trees, uncover health risks, and discover ancestral connections in ways that were once unimaginable.

For many people, these DNA tests offer fascinating insights into their family history, but for donor-conceived individuals, these tests represent a new era of truth-telling. For someone who has been told they were conceived using a sperm or egg donor, taking one of these tests can sometimes lead to an unexpected—and potentially life-changing—revelation. These tests may uncover biological relatives who were previously unknown, including half-siblings or even the biological parent, if the donor's identity is not anonymous.

With the vast number of users on platforms like Ancestry.com and 23andMe, the likelihood of uncovering unexpected family connections is higher than ever. People who take these tests often find themselves connected to genetic relatives they never knew existed. For a donor-conceived person, this could mean connecting with a donor sibling, or in rare cases, even discovering the identity of their biological parent.

These revelations can be a powerful tool for self-discovery. Learning about biological family members can offer a deeper understanding of one's genetic traits, health risks, and heritage. However, these discoveries can also come with emotional challenges, especially if the individual was not prepared for the new information or if the truth contradicts the family narrative they grew up with.

For example, a donor-conceived child might take a DNA test and, through the results, learn that they have a half-sibling they were not previously told about. This can be an exhilarating and sometimes overwhelming experience, particularly if the sibling is discovered through a match on a genetic testing site and the two individuals begin communicating. This type of discovery can raise complex questions about family relationships, identity, and belonging.

In some cases, a child may even find that the biological parent is not the anonymous donor they were told about, but rather a person they have no direct connection with. This can lead to a range of emotions, from joy at finding a biological parent to confusion, loss, and a sense of betrayal. The possibility of reconnecting with biological family members can open up new opportunities for connection and understanding, but it can also be fraught with emotional challenges.

Stories of Sudden Reveals and Reunions

The stories of individuals who have experienced sudden revelations through genetic testing are both compelling and poignant. Take, for example, the story of Emma, a young woman who grew up knowing she was donor-conceived, but whose family had always maintained that her donor was anonymous. She decided to take a 23andMe test to learn more about her heritage and possibly connect with distant relatives. To her surprise, she discovered a close genetic match—a man who was identified as her half-brother.

Emma's first reaction was one of disbelief, followed by excitement and curiosity. She contacted her half-brother through the platform and began a conversation that led to the discovery of a complex and emotional family history. Emma learned that her biological father had been a sperm donor in the early 1990s, but he had also maintained contact with some of his biological children, including her half-brother, whom she had never met.

The reunion with her half-brother brought both joy and a sense of closure, as Emma had always felt there was something missing from her identity. However, the emotional journey was not without its challenges. Emma had to navigate her feelings of connection to her social parents, whom she loved deeply, and the complex reality of being connected to someone she had never met. There was also a sense of guilt and anxiety about how her social parents might react to the discovery, as the family had always maintained that the donor was anonymous and that Emma had no further connections to her biological roots.

For other individuals, the process of uncovering unexpected family members is not always so smooth or celebratory. Some donor-conceived people who discover genetic relatives through DNA testing may feel overwhelmed by the flood of new information. They may experience feelings of confusion about their place in the family, questions about the truth they were told about their origins, or even a sense of loss about not having known their biological family.

The discovery of genetic relatives can also stir up deep emotional responses for parents who may not have been prepared for their child to uncover these truths. Parents might feel betrayed, guilty, or anxious about the new reality that their child's family narrative has changed. These emotional responses can complicate the process of integrating new family members into the child's life.

As the stories of sudden reveals and reunions show, DNA testing has introduced a new complexity to the experience of identity. The truth is not always what people expect, and while some discoveries may lead to joy and connection, others may spark confusion, tension, or even a sense of loss. The emotional and psychological impacts of these revelations are profound and require careful consideration, especially when they happen unexpectedly.

Section 2: Empowering Instead of Panicking

How to Support Kids Who Discover Unexpected Roots

As DNA testing becomes more common, it is increasingly likely that donor-conceived children will come across unexpected family connections. For parents, the prospect of their child discovering the truth through a genetic test can be anxiety-provoking, but it is crucial to remember that these discoveries can be empowering if handled with care and empathy.

Supporting a child who discovers unexpected roots begins with acknowledging the emotional complexity of the situation. The first step is to listen. The child will likely have a range of emotions upon discovering new family members, and it's important to provide a safe space for them to express their feelings without fear of judgment. Whether they feel joy, confusion, anger, or sadness, these emotions are valid and should be respected.

Validate their feelings: It's crucial to validate the child's experience by acknowledging the impact of the discovery. Saying something like, "I understand this is a lot to process, and it's okay to have mixed feelings about it," can go a long way in helping the child feel supported. It's also helpful to reassure them that they are loved and that their place in the family is secure. Parents should emphasize that their relationship with the child has not changed and that this discovery does not affect their bond.

Encourage open communication: It is essential to keep the lines of communication open with the child, especially if they want to explore the newfound connections. Whether they wish to reach out to a biological sibling or even meet a biological parent, parents should allow the child to take the lead in these interactions while providing guidance and support.

Seek professional guidance: In some cases, it may be beneficial to involve a therapist or counselor, especially if the child is struggling with complex emotions or if the discovery has caused significant distress. A professional can help the child process their feelings and offer strategies for coping with the emotional challenges that arise from discovering unexpected roots.

Legal, Emotional, and Practical Next Steps

The emotional journey of discovering unexpected family connections is only one part of the equation. There are also legal and practical considerations to keep in mind. Depending on the jurisdiction and the laws surrounding donor conception, there may be legal steps to take in order to formalize any newfound relationships or clarify the child's legal status in relation to their biological family.

Legal considerations: In some places, laws regarding the rights of donor-conceived individuals vary significantly. For example, in countries where anonymous donation is prohibited, the donor may be legally required to disclose their identity to the child once they reach adulthood. In other places, legal agreements may exist that protect the anonymity of the donor and limit the child's ability to access genetic information. Parents should educate themselves about the legal rights of their child and any steps they may need to take to ensure that the child's rights are respected in the context of their biological family.

Practical considerations: As the child navigates their relationships with new genetic relatives, parents may need to consider how these relationships fit into the family's dynamics. For example, if the child wishes to meet a half-sibling or biological parent, parents should approach these meetings with care and preparation. It may be necessary to establish boundaries and expectations for these relationships to ensure that the child feels safe and secure as they navigate their evolving sense of identity.

Emotional support: Throughout this process, parents should continue to provide emotional support and reaffirm the importance of the family unit. While discovering new family members can be an exciting and enriching experience, it can also bring up feelings of insecurity or confusion. It's important to emphasize that the child's place in the family is unshakable and that these new discoveries do not change the love and connection they share with their parents.

Conclusion

The advent of DNA testing has introduced new complexities in the lives of donor-conceived children, offering both opportunities for discovery and challenges for identity formation. While these tests have made it easier to connect with biological relatives, they also present the potential for accidental truths and emotional upheaval. The stories of sudden reveals and reunions illustrate the profound impact that these discoveries can have on a child's sense of self and their relationship with their family.

As DNA tests become increasingly commonplace, it is crucial for parents to be prepared to support their children through unexpected revelations. By fostering open communication, validating emotions, and providing legal and practical guidance, parents can help their children navigate the complexities of newfound biological connections with confidence and security. In a world where the truth about one's origins can be just a DNA test away, offering unconditional love and support remains the cornerstone of helping children build strong, integrated identities.

Chapter 6

Talking About the Donor (Without a Biography)

Introduction:

The conversation surrounding donor conception can be complex, and one of the most challenging aspects for parents is discussing the donor with their children. For many families, the donor may be anonymous or only known through sparse, clinical details. Yet, the question remains: how do we talk about someone who is, in many ways, a stranger to the child but who still plays a fundamental role in their genetic makeup? In some cases, the donor may be reachable or known, presenting additional complexities when navigating how much information to share and when.

This chapter explores how to create a meaningful donor narrative, even when the details are limited or nonexistent. In Section 1, we will examine the importance of creating a donor narrative that respects the child's need for identity while avoiding idealization or demonization of the donor figure. In Section 2, we will delve into what happens when the donor is known or reachable, offering strategies for managing expectations, contact, and the emotional dynamics that come with navigating this connection. Whether the donor is a mysterious figure or a known presence, talking about them thoughtfully and responsibly is crucial for the child's emotional well-being and sense of self.

Section 1: The Myth, the Mystery, the Person

Creating a Donor Narrative When Details Are Sparse

For many donor-conceived children, the donor is an elusive figure. In the case of anonymous donation, details about the donor may be extremely limited, often consisting of only a few facts such as age, profession, education, and health history. While these details can help frame a basic understanding of the donor's background, they may not offer much insight into the person behind the genetic contribution. Yet, even in the absence of a rich biography, it's important to find a way to create a meaningful narrative that helps the child understand their biological roots in a way that is both positive and empowering.

The first key to creating a donor narrative is to frame the donor's role in a way that emphasizes their importance without making them the central figure in the child's life. A donor is, after all, just one part of a much larger story—a story that includes the social and emotional ties that bind the child to their parents, family, and community. The donor, even if unknown or mysterious, played a significant part in the child's creation, but it is the child's relationship with their social parents and their wider family that provides the foundation of their identity. It's essential to present the donor's role in a neutral light—without elevating them into a larger-than-life figure, but also without reducing their importance to a mere biological detail.

When creating a donor narrative, parents should be cautious of both idealizing and demonizing the donor. Idealization often occurs when the donor is viewed as an almost perfect figure—someone who embodies all of the child's hopes, dreams, and desires. In contrast, demonization might happen if the donor is seen as a shadowy, negative presence—someone who is distant, anonymous, or even morally questionable. Both approaches can have negative emotional consequences for the child.

If a child learns about their donor through an idealized narrative, they may develop unrealistic expectations about who the donor is and what they represent. They might imagine the donor as someone who is perfect in every way—perhaps a brilliant scientist, a beautiful artist, or a beloved hero in some sense. This idealized image can lead to disappointment or confusion if the child ever learns more about the donor or attempts to form a real relationship with them. The child may feel as if they do not measure up to the donor's imagined qualities or that their connection with the donor is somehow incomplete or unfulfilling.

On the other hand, if the donor is demonized or portrayed as an absent or uncaring figure, the child may internalize feelings of abandonment or inadequacy. They may grow up resenting the donor or viewing their biological origins as a source of shame or emotional deprivation. This can lead to an unhealthy view of their identity and a negative self-concept, which can undermine their emotional development and their ability to form positive relationships in the future.

Rather than relying on idealization or demonization, a more balanced approach is needed—one that focuses on the donor's role as part of the child's larger story but does not elevate or diminish their importance. A neutral narrative that includes the facts without embellishing or distorting them allows the child to form their own understanding of the donor, one that is based on reality rather than fantasy.

Parents can use this neutral narrative to emphasize that the donor's role is part of the child's unique story—neither good nor bad, but simply part of who they are. For instance, parents might say: "Your donor was a person who helped us bring you into the world, and we are grateful for that. We don't know everything about them, but we do know that they gave us a great gift. And what's most important is that you are loved and cherished by us and your family."

This narrative emphasizes gratitude and acceptance, framing the donor's role as important but not central to the child's entire identity. It also leaves space for the child to ask questions and explore their feelings about the donor in their own time, rather than imposing a rigid narrative that they might feel pressured to accept.

Avoiding Idealization or Demonization

As we mentioned earlier, the most important challenge when creating a donor narrative is avoiding the extremes of idealization or demonization. Both extremes can be damaging in different ways.

Idealization: Idealizing the donor can create unrealistic expectations and may contribute to feelings of disappointment later. If the donor is placed on a pedestal—viewed as an almost mythical figure—the child may come to expect that a relationship with the donor will fulfill all of their emotional needs, or they may develop an inflated sense of self-importance based on the perceived brilliance or beauty of the donor. This can lead to a sense of inadequacy if the child feels that they cannot live up to the idealized image of the donor.

Parents should strive to present the donor as a human being—someone who made an important contribution, but who is not a perfect or faultless figure. The donor is, after all, just one piece of the puzzle, and while they played a crucial role in the child's biological makeup, they are not the sole determinant of who the child is. Parents should emphasize that the child's worth is not tied to the donor's perceived perfection but to their own intrinsic qualities and the love and support they receive from their family.

Demonization: On the other hand, demonizing the donor can create negative feelings of abandonment, confusion, or even anger. If the donor is seen as an uncaring or even morally questionable figure, the child may internalize those negative feelings. This can lead to a fractured sense of self, as the child may feel that they are somehow tainted or incomplete because of their biological origins.

To avoid this, it is important to present the donor's role in neutral terms, emphasizing the fact that their biological contribution does not define the child's worth. Parents can frame the donor's role as one part of the story, rather than placing judgment on their character or actions. For example, parents can say, "Your donor was a person who helped us become a family. We don't know much about them, but what we know is that you are our child, and you are loved no matter what."

This narrative approach helps prevent the child from feeling that their biological origins are something to be ashamed of or rejected. Instead, it affirms the child's place in the family and their right to feel valued, regardless of their donor's history or identity.

Section 2: When the Donor is Known or Reachable

Managing Expectations and Contact

In cases where the donor is known or even reachable, the dynamic of talking about the donor becomes more complex. In these situations, it is essential to manage the child's expectations, as well as the parents' expectations, about what a relationship with the donor might look like.

When the donor is known, it can be tempting to imagine an idealized reunion or relationship. The child may have an overwhelming desire to meet the donor or form a connection, believing that this person holds the key to understanding themselves better. It is important, however, to acknowledge that while a relationship with the donor may offer valuable insights, it may not provide all the answers the child is seeking. In many cases, the donor may not be interested in maintaining an ongoing relationship or may have different emotional or practical reasons for keeping their distance.

Managing expectations is crucial in these situations. Parents should talk openly with the child about what contact with the donor might entail and what it may not provide. For instance, the donor may be open to meeting the child but may not want a full-fledged relationship. They may be willing to provide medical history or answer questions, but they may not want to take on a parental role. By managing the child's expectations from the beginning, parents can help prevent potential disappointment and emotional distress.

Navigating Boundaries, Curiosity, and Emotions

If the donor is reachable or willing to engage, it's essential to navigate boundaries carefully. The child's curiosity about their biological parent is natural, but it's important to establish clear and respectful boundaries to ensure that everyone involved feels comfortable and respected. Parents should help the child understand that the donor is a person with their own life, circumstances, and emotional boundaries. The donor may not want to be involved in every aspect of the child's life, and that decision should be respected.

Equally important is the emotional dimension of these connections. Meeting the donor or learning more about them can trigger a wide range of emotions for both the child and the parents. The child may feel a deep sense of connection, or they may feel overwhelmed, confused, or disappointed if the relationship does not meet their expectations. Parents should be prepared to offer support as the child processes these emotions. Whether the contact is brief or ongoing, parents must reaffirm the child's sense of self-worth and emphasize that the love and support they provide is not contingent upon the donor's involvement.

Emotional check-ins should become a regular part of the process. Whether the child is considering reaching out to the donor, meeting them in person, or simply asking more questions about their background, parents should provide a safe space for the child to express their feelings and concerns. By doing so, parents help the child navigate the complexities of these relationships with empathy, compassion, and emotional clarity.

Conclusion

Talking about the donor, whether they are a mysterious figure or a known presence, is an essential part of helping donor-conceived children build a healthy and integrated sense of identity. Creating a balanced donor narrative—one that avoids idealization and demonization—helps the child understand their origins in a way that is empowering and realistic. When the donor is known or reachable, managing expectations, respecting boundaries, and supporting emotional exploration are key to ensuring that these connections enhance the child's sense of self without overshadowing their relationships with their social family. By approaching the topic with care, respect, and openness, parents can help their children navigate the complexities of donor conception with confidence and emotional resilience.

Chapter 7

The Family Mirror: Parents, Siblings, and Reflection

Introduction:

Family dynamics are shaped by more than just biology; they are built on love, care, and shared experiences. For donor-conceived children, the concept of family takes on a unique complexity, as the biological connection may be partial or unknown. Yet, despite the intricacies of their origins, these children often share powerful, enduring bonds with their social parents and siblings. The family unit becomes the mirror through which the child reflects on who they are, their sense of belonging, and their role in the world.

This chapter explores the concept of family in the context of donor conception, with particular focus on the relationships that help children form their identities. In Section 1, we dive into the bond between social parents and children, emphasizing how love and attachment, rather than biological ties, are the cornerstone of a secure and healthy relationship. We will also explore how to respond to questions like, "Are you my real mom/dad?" with confidence and empathy. In Section 2, we expand the discussion to include siblings, both biological and half-siblings, exploring the impact of same-donor networks, DNA connections, and the complex web of identity that comes with discovering genetic relatives. We will look at the emotional journey that siblings navigate—ranging from deep connection to rejection—and how these relationships evolve within the context of donor conception.

Section 1: The Social Parent Bond

Love Over Biology: The Science of Secure Attachment

For donor-conceived children, the relationship with their social parents—the individuals who raise them, love them, and care for them— is the central bond that shapes their sense of self. While biological connections can play a role in identity, it is the love and support provided by social parents that truly defines family for most children. This concept is grounded in attachment theory, which emphasizes the importance of early, consistent caregiving in the development of secure emotional bonds.

Attachment theory, first developed by John Bowlby, posits that children need a strong, dependable relationship with a primary caregiver to feel secure and develop healthy emotional regulation. This secure attachment forms the basis of a child's ability to explore the world, form relationships with others, and develop a healthy sense of self-worth. Secure attachment is not determined by biology, but by the presence of a caregiver who is attuned to the child's needs and who provides comfort, love, and stability. For donor-conceived children, their social parents serve as these primary caregivers, offering the nurturing environment that helps the child grow into a confident, emotionally secure individual.

The concept of love over biology is fundamental for understanding how donor-conceived children bond with their parents. The idea that love, care, and emotional connection are more important than genetic ties is critical in ensuring that these children develop healthy, integrated identities. In many ways, a child's emotional attachment to their social parents is the lens through which they view the world and their place in it. This attachment doesn't diminish their need for information about their biological origins, but it anchors them firmly in the emotional reality of being loved and cared for by the people they call family.

For parents, fostering this secure attachment involves being responsive to the child's needs, offering consistent love, and creating an environment where the child feels safe and valued. This includes both the physical and emotional aspects of caregiving—such as being present, providing comfort during times of distress, and creating positive, nurturing experiences. Research shows that children who feel securely attached to their parents are more likely to develop healthy relationships later in life, experience greater emotional stability, and have a positive sense of self.

Answering "Are You My Real Mom/Dad?" With Confidence

At some point in their development, many donor-conceived children will ask the question, "Are you my real mom/dad?" This question often arises as children begin to make sense of the world around them and notice differences between themselves and others, especially as they encounter new information about their biological origins. It is natural for children to wonder about their connections to the people around them, and this question is not a challenge to the legitimacy of the parental bond, but rather an inquiry into how family is defined.

For social parents, answering this question with confidence is critical to ensuring that the child feels secure and loved. The answer should reinforce the idea that the social parents are the child's "real" parents, regardless of their biological connection. This doesn't diminish the child's need to know about their donor origins, but it affirms that the parent-child bond is not defined by genetics but by the emotional and social relationship they share.

A confident, affirming response to this question might sound something like: "Yes, I am your real mom/dad. I may not be your biological parent, but I am your parent in every way that matters. I love you with all my heart, and nothing will ever change that." This answer reinforces the importance of the social parent-child relationship and emphasizes that being a "real" parent is about emotional connection, love, and commitment, not genetics.

It's also important to acknowledge the child's curiosity about their biological origins without undermining the strength of the parent-child bond. For example, a parent could add, "I know you're curious about your donor, and I'm here to help you understand where you come from. But know that I will always be here for you, and that will never change." This response validates the child's need to explore their biological roots while maintaining the security and stability of the relationship with the social parents.

The key is to approach these conversations with confidence and reassurance, helping the child understand that their value is not contingent upon their biological relationship with their parents, but rather on the love and care they receive. This kind of conversation reinforces the idea that being a family is about emotional connection, mutual support, and shared history, not simply genetic links.

Section 2: Siblings and Same-Donor Networks

DNA Siblings, Half-Siblings, and Identity Webs

When donor-conceived children begin to learn about their biological origins, they often discover that they have siblings, either through the same donor or through genetic relatives. These siblings may be referred to as DNA siblings or half-siblings, depending on whether they share one or both biological parents. The concept of DNA siblings can be particularly significant for donor-conceived children, as it offers an opportunity to form connections with people who share some of their genetic makeup, even if they were raised in different families.

For many donor-conceived children, discovering DNA siblings is an exciting and emotional experience. These newfound siblings can provide a sense of connection and shared history, especially if the child has felt a sense of disconnection from their biological roots. For some, meeting a half-sibling may help them feel more whole, as it provides the opportunity to see physical similarities and share experiences with someone who has the same biological heritage.

However, these relationships can also be complicated by the varying degrees of involvement, emotional connection, and personal history. Half-siblings may have different family dynamics, or they may not have been raised with the same cultural or emotional values. The discovery of a DNA sibling may lead to feelings of curiosity, excitement, or anxiety, and the emotional journey of connecting with half-siblings can vary widely from one individual to another.

In some cases, donor-conceived individuals might also connect with same-donor networks, where people who were conceived through the same donor find each other through online databases, social media groups, or even genetic testing services. These networks can create a powerful sense of community and belonging, as individuals learn that they share a biological connection with others. For some, these networks can provide an opportunity to explore their genetic heritage more deeply, sharing experiences and learning from others who are in similar situations.

The concept of identity webs becomes relevant in this context, as the donor-conceived child begins to form an understanding of themselves in relation to their biological and social family. These identity webs are built through interactions with both social and genetic family members, creating a multifaceted understanding of who the child is. The more connections a child forms—whether through DNA siblings, half-siblings, or same-donor networks—the more the child's sense of self expands, incorporating both biological and social dimensions.

Connection, Rejection, and Everything In Between

While some donor-conceived individuals form close, lasting connections with their DNA siblings, others may experience feelings of rejection, confusion, or discomfort. The emotional journey of discovering half-siblings can be unpredictable, as the child navigates new relationships and tries to make sense of the familial bond they share with these individuals.

Connection can occur when siblings feel a sense of commonality, shared experience, or emotional closeness. The shared experience of being donor-conceived can create an instant bond, as both parties may have similar feelings about their biological origins. The physical resemblance between siblings—such as shared facial features, mannerisms, or even health conditions—can deepen the sense of connection. In some cases, siblings may choose to meet in person, creating lasting relationships that extend beyond the biological link.

However, rejection can also be a part of the process. Some donor-conceived children may struggle to accept the presence of new siblings, especially if they feel that these relationships interfere with the family dynamics they have known. They may feel uncomfortable with the idea of sharing their biological origins with someone they've never met or may fear that the new sibling will change their relationship with their parents. Rejection can also occur if the other sibling or family members are not interested in forming a relationship or if the connection feels forced or awkward.

Everything in between is equally possible. The emotional complexity of sibling relationships in the context of donor conception is unique, and each experience will be different. Some donor-conceived children may feel an overwhelming sense of connection upon meeting a half-sibling, while others may struggle with feelings of confusion or disorientation. The process of building relationships with DNA siblings is fluid, and it may require time, patience, and emotional support.

Parents can help navigate these complex dynamics by encouraging open communication, setting healthy boundaries, and being empathetic to the child's emotional responses. They should also allow the child to take the lead in how they wish to engage with their DNA siblings, offering guidance and support as needed but allowing the child to form their own relationships at their own pace.

Conclusion

The family dynamics of donor-conceived children are shaped not just by biological connections but by the love, care, and support provided by social parents and the relationships they build with siblings, both biological and non-biological. For social parents, fostering a secure attachment with their child is the foundation of a strong, healthy bond, while offering responses that affirm the parent-child relationship can help address questions about biological connections with confidence.

For siblings, both genetic and non-genetic, the process of discovery is often filled with a mix of excitement, confusion, and emotional complexity. Whether through DNA siblings or same-donor networks, the child's sense of identity expands as they explore these relationships.

By approaching these connections with patience, empathy, and open communication, parents can help their child navigate the evolving web of relationships and build a sense of self that honors both their biological and social family.

Chapter 8

Emotional Milestones and Vulnerable Ages

Introduction:

Every child's emotional journey is unique, and for those conceived through sperm or egg donation, the path to self-discovery can be complex. While the stages of emotional growth for donor-conceived children parallel those of all children—curiosity in early childhood, questioning during adolescence, and a search for identity in the teen years—the emotional milestones they encounter often come with additional layers. These children may navigate the intricate terrain of understanding their biological roots, reconciling their family structure, and seeking a sense of belonging. From their first realizations of difference to their adolescent search for wholeness, donor-conceived children go through a series of emotional shifts that, while natural, are often marked by vulnerability.

This chapter delves into the emotional milestones and struggles that donor-conceived children experience as they grow, offering insights into how their identities evolve throughout childhood and adolescence. In Section 1, we will explore how their understanding of self-changes through the toddler, tween, and teen years, each stage marked by new questions, new awareness, and new emotional needs. In Section 2, we will identify emotional red flags—signs that a child may be struggling with shame, anger, anxiety, or feelings of not belonging—and provide guidance on when to seek professional help. Understanding these emotional milestones is key to providing the right support at the right time, ensuring that donor-conceived children can form a secure, positive identity.

Section 1: Identity Shifts Through Childhood

Toddlers: Seeds of Difference

The toddler years are a time when children begin to develop a sense of themselves as separate individuals. They start to notice the world around them and understand their place within it. For most children, this is the age when they first begin to perceive differences in appearance, behavior, or family structure. While the idea of biological origins may not be fully developed, toddlers often begin to notice small things—such as their physical traits or the ways they might differ from their parents or peers—that subtly plant the seeds of difference.

At this age, children are still forming their early concepts of identity. They may observe physical characteristics that set them apart from their social parents, such as skin tone, hair color, or eye shape. This recognition is typically innocent and not accompanied by any deep reflection, but it's a significant developmental moment. Toddlers may ask questions like, "Why do I look different from you?" or "How did I get here?" These questions are typically not loaded with anxiety or confusion, but they reflect the beginning of a child's cognitive development in terms of their awareness of self and others.

For donor-conceived children, these observations can mark the beginning of their understanding of biological difference. At this stage, toddlers are more likely to notice that they don't share physical characteristics with their parents, but they might not yet understand the significance of these differences. This is the "seed stage"—the early beginnings of a child's curiosity about family and origins. While they won't fully comprehend the concept of donor conception, they may begin to sense that their family story is unique.

How parents respond during this stage is critical. Even though toddlers may not have the capacity to understand complex ideas about genetics, it's still important to introduce simple, age-appropriate concepts about family and origins. A gentle and positive approach can help set the tone for future conversations. A parent might say, "You were born with help from a very special person who gave us the gift of life." This framing is simple but positive, setting the foundation for deeper conversations as the child grows older.

While the questions toddlers ask are often simple, the emotional undercurrent is significant. This is a time when parents must reinforce the idea that the child is loved and accepted, regardless of biological connections. The child's sense of self at this stage is rooted in their primary attachment to their parents and caregivers, and this attachment becomes the foundation for their later emotional development.

Tweens: Questioning and Awareness

As children enter the tween years (ages 9-12), they begin to develop a more sophisticated understanding of the world around them. This is a time of increasing self-awareness, curiosity, and emotional complexity. For donor-conceived children, the tween years often mark the beginning of deeper questions about their origins. They may start to recognize more clearly that their family structure is different from those of their peers.

During this stage, tweens begin to understand the concepts of biology and genetics. They may start to realize that there is a biological parent they do not know, and the awareness of this "difference" becomes more pronounced. The child may notice that they don't look like their social parents, or they may observe that their friends' families seem more similar to each other in physical traits and family structure. These realizations can lead to more pointed questions about their origins, such as, "Why don't I look like you?" or "Where did I come from?"

At this point, the child is entering a phase where they are exploring their identity more consciously. They are beginning to distinguish themselves from their parents, peers, and others, and they may start to ask questions about how their family fits into the larger societal picture. In some cases, they may experience confusion or curiosity about their biological roots. This stage is one of emerging self-awareness—where the child becomes more conscious of who they are and how they fit into the world. It's a period of growing emotional complexity as they begin to question their place in the family and society.

For donor-conceived children, this awareness often sparks an emotional need to learn more about their donor, particularly if they feel the absence of biological resemblance to their social parents. The child may not fully understand why they feel this way, but they might begin to experience a sense of missing something in their story. The emotional reaction could range from curiosity to frustration, as the child grapples with the unknown aspects of their identity.

Parents play a vital role in supporting their child through this questioning phase. It's important to provide truthful, age-appropriate information, while also acknowledging the child's emotional experience. This is a time when parents can start to introduce more details about the donor, answering questions with openness and honesty. However, it's equally important to emphasize that the child's worth and identity are not determined solely by genetics. Parents should continue to reassure the child that they are loved and valued for who they are, irrespective of their biological background.

Tweens may also begin to compare themselves more with others, which can bring up feelings of difference or alienation. This can be exacerbated for donor-conceived children if they are the only one in their social group with a non-traditional family structure. It's crucial for parents to be aware of these feelings and to offer support as the child navigates these new emotional complexities.

Teens: Searching for Wholeness

The teenage years are marked by a profound search for identity. Adolescence is a time when the child's sense of self becomes increasingly influenced by their peers, their social roles, and their desire to understand their own uniqueness. For donor-conceived children, this period of identity exploration is often intensified by the complex process of reconciling their biological origins with their sense of belonging to their family.

During adolescence, teens are more likely to question the very fabric of their identity. For donor-conceived teens, this may involve questions such as, "Who am I really?" and "How do I fit into my family?" The search for wholeness during this period involves not only a desire to understand their biological origins but also a deeper quest for connection and belonging. Teens often begin to feel the absence of biological ties more keenly, and may seek out more information about their donor or explore the possibility of connecting with biological relatives.

At this stage, the emotional landscape is one of complexity. Donor-conceived teens may feel a mixture of curiosity, excitement, and frustration as they explore their biological roots. They may long for a sense of connection to someone who shares their physical traits, personality, or family history. This search for wholeness can sometimes lead to feelings of alienation, particularly if the teen feels disconnected from their donor or if they have not had the opportunity to meet or learn about biological family members.

The process of identity exploration during adolescence often involves an increased emotional investment in understanding one's biological heritage. This can be especially true if the teen feels a lack of information or connection to their donor. For some teens, the desire to connect with biological relatives can feel like an overwhelming need to "complete" themselves or to understand who they are in a more profound way.

While this process of searching for wholeness is a normal part of adolescent development, it can sometimes lead to confusion, frustration, or even resentment. Teens may feel like they are missing a crucial part of their story, and this can contribute to a sense of disconnection or dissatisfaction. Parents must be sensitive to these emotional shifts and provide guidance and reassurance during this search for identity.

The emotional struggles teens face around donor conception are often tied to the broader issues of autonomy, identity, and independence. Teens are in the process of differentiating themselves from their parents, and this process may intensify if they feel different due to their biological origins. Parents can help support their teen by fostering open communication and validating their emotional experiences. It's important to encourage the teen to explore their identity in a way that feels authentic to them, while also reinforcing the strength of their relationship with their social parents.

Section 2: Emotional Red Flags

Shame, Anger, Anxiety, and Belonging Struggles

While identity exploration is a natural and necessary part of growing up, donor-conceived children may experience certain emotional struggles as they process their origins. Emotional red flags, such as shame, anger, anxiety, and belonging struggles, can indicate that the child is struggling with their identity and their sense of connection to their family and biological roots.

- **Shame**: Donor-conceived children may experience feelings of shame, particularly if they have internalized the idea that being conceived through donor sperm or egg is somehow different or less than other ways of being born. Shame can also arise if the child feels that their family's story is secret or hidden, or if they perceive themselves as different from their peers in ways that make them feel inadequate. Shame can be insidious, affecting the child's self-worth and sense of belonging.

- **Anger**: Anger is another common emotional response, particularly for teens. They may feel angry at the donor for being absent or not a part of their lives. Anger can also be directed toward the social parents for keeping the donor's identity hidden or for not providing enough information. Adolescents in particular may experience frustration or anger about not having control over their own family story and may express feelings of resentment about being donor-conceived.

- **Anxiety**: Anxiety often arises when the child feels uncertain or overwhelmed by questions about their origins. The unknowns about their biological roots can lead to a sense of anxiety about identity and belonging. This anxiety may manifest as a fear of rejection, worry about meeting the donor or donor siblings, or concerns about how their family will react to new information.

Anxiety can also emerge during periods of transition, such as adolescence, when the child's sense of self is being reshaped.

- **Belonging Struggles**: A sense of not fully belonging—whether within their family, social group, or the world at large—is a common emotional struggle for donor-conceived children. Teens, in particular, may feel alienated if they are the only ones in their peer group with a non-traditional family structure. These feelings can be compounded by the search for identity and the desire to understand their place in the family and in society.

When to Seek Professional Help

It's crucial to recognize when a donor-conceived child is struggling with emotional challenges that go beyond normal developmental milestones. Prolonged or intense emotional struggles, such as persistent shame, anger, anxiety, or feelings of not belonging, can interfere with the child's ability to form a healthy identity. If these emotional issues persist or intensify, it may be time to seek professional help.

Parents should consider professional guidance if:

- The child exhibits signs of depression or prolonged sadness that interfere with their daily life.

- There is increased anger or acting out that seems linked to their donor conception or family dynamics.

- The child expresses anxiety about their identity or biological origins in ways that affect their social relationships or self-esteem.

- The child has difficulty forming relationships or experiences a deep sense of disconnection or alienation from others.

Therapists who specialize in identity development, family dynamics, or issues related to donor conception can be incredibly helpful in supporting both the child and the family. Therapy provides a safe space for children to process their emotions, explore their identity, and work through any issues related to their donor conception. Family therapy can also be beneficial, as it helps to foster open communication, resolve conflicts, and build stronger emotional bonds within the family unit.

Conclusion

The emotional milestones of donor-conceived children are intricately tied to their understanding of themselves, their family, and their biological origins. From the toddler years, when seeds of difference are first planted, to the tween and teen years, when identity exploration intensifies, donor-conceived children experience a series of emotional shifts that shape their sense of self. While these emotional challenges are a normal part of growing up, they can also bring struggles such as shame, anger, anxiety, and belonging difficulties. Parents play a critical role in supporting their child's emotional development, and recognizing the emotional red flags is essential for ensuring the child's well-being. By providing open communication, fostering a strong sense of belonging, and seeking professional help when necessary, parents can guide their child through these emotional milestones and help them build a strong, positive identity.

Chapter 9

Culture, Community, and Representation

Introduction:

Culture and community shape our understanding of identity, belonging, and how we see ourselves in the world. For donor-conceived children, the process of forming their identity is shaped not only by their family but also by how they are represented in the broader culture. Growing up in a world where narratives around family are often defined by traditional biological ties can leave these children searching for reflections of themselves in the stories and characters around them. Representation matters—it shapes how children view themselves and their place in society.

In this chapter, we will explore how donor-conceived children navigate their sense of self in a world that may not always reflect their experiences. Section 1 focuses on the importance of representation in media, books, and everyday conversations. We will discuss the need for donor-conceived characters and stories that normalize difference, highlighting the impact of seeing oneself in the world around them. In Section 2, we turn to the social sphere, where donor-conceived children must navigate curiosity and sometimes insensitive questions from peers. We'll examine how to create supportive environments in schools, among friends, and in other social settings, and explore how to build safe circles of allies who foster understanding and acceptance.

Section 1: Seeing Yourself in the World

The Need for Donor-Conceived Characters and Stories

When it comes to identity formation, one of the most powerful tools for children is the ability to see themselves reflected in the stories, media, and characters they encounter. Representation is critical—it helps children understand that their experiences are valid and that they are not alone. For donor-conceived children, however, this representation is often lacking or misrepresented. Mainstream narratives of family and identity typically center around biological connections, which can leave these children struggling to find characters or stories they can truly identify with.

In literature, television, and film, family structures are often presented as traditional, with biological ties being the norm. The absence of donor-conceived characters in mainstream media reinforces the notion that their family structures are not "normal" or are somehow outside the norm. This lack of representation can leave donor-conceived children feeling marginalized, isolated, or confused about their place in the broader narrative of what it means to be a family.

There is a growing need for donor-conceived characters in books, TV shows, and films who reflect the realities of modern family structures. Just as children benefit from seeing diverse cultural, racial, and gender representations, donor-conceived children also need to see stories that reflect their experiences. These stories should show the complexities of their family dynamics, the relationships they have with their social parents, and the sometimes intricate connections they may have with their biological roots.

Donor-conceived children need to see characters who, like them, may not share the same genetic material as their parents but who experience love, identity struggles, and belonging in ways that resonate with their own lives. These characters can help normalize their experiences and provide a sense of validation. Stories that feature donor-conceived characters can also explore the nuances of being raised by social parents while grappling with questions of biological origins, making the experience relatable and empowering for children going through similar journeys.

In addition to storytelling in media, it's essential for parents, caregivers, and educators to create narratives in their everyday conversations that validate the experiences of donor-conceived children. Simple phrases like, "Every family is different, and that's what makes each one special," or "What matters most is the love and care we share with each other," help to reinforce the idea that donor conception is just one way of creating a family, and it's just as valid and important as any other family structure.

Normalizing Difference in Books, TV, and Conversations

Normalizing difference is key to ensuring that donor-conceived children don't feel isolated or "othered." When children grow up seeing their unique family structure as just another normal variation of family, they are more likely to develop a healthy sense of self and belonging. The absence of donor-conceived families in mainstream media can perpetuate feelings of shame or confusion. However, when donor-conceived characters appear in books, TV shows, and movies, they provide a positive model for children to identify with, reducing the stigma often associated with being different.

One way to normalize difference is through diverse representation in children's literature. Books that feature donor-conceived children as protagonists or part of the family unit help children see that their experiences are shared by others, both in fiction and in real life. These stories should reflect a wide range of family dynamics, showing not only donor-conceived children who know their donor but also those who may be searching for their biological roots or exploring the complexities of their identity.

Television and film, too, play a vital role in shaping how children see themselves and their families. While there has been progress in recent years with the portrayal of diverse family structures, including same-sex parents, blended families, and adoptive families, there remains a notable absence of donor-conceived families in mainstream media. Creating TV shows or movies that portray donor-conceived families as normal, loving, and fully integrated into society is essential to fostering inclusivity. The inclusion of these characters will also encourage empathy among non-donor-conceived children, teaching them about diversity in family structures and the importance of acceptance.

Beyond fictional stories, it is also important to integrate conversations about donor conception into everyday dialogue. Parents and educators can help normalize the experience by acknowledging that many children have diverse family backgrounds. This can be done casually, for example, by including donor-conceived characters in classroom activities or in discussions about family diversity. Even mentioning that some children have parents who are not genetically related to them can help foster an environment of acceptance and understanding.

By normalizing these conversations, we give donor-conceived children permission to talk about their family stories and biological origins without fear of judgment. It also helps the broader community—friends, family members, and peers—understand that these children are just like any other, deserving of love, respect, and acceptance.

Section 2: School, Friends, and Social Settings

Navigating Curiosity and Insensitive Questions

As donor-conceived children grow older and interact with their peers, they may encounter questions about their family that can be uncomfortable or intrusive. Curiosity is a natural part of childhood, and children often ask questions about the differences they observe in others, including family structures. While curiosity is understandable, sometimes children (and even adults) ask questions that can be insensitive or even hurtful.

Questions like, "Who's your real dad?" or "Why don't you look like your parents?" may seem innocent on the surface, but they can cause donor-conceived children to feel like they don't belong or are somehow "less than" their peers. These questions can be especially difficult if the child hasn't fully processed their own feelings about being donor-conceived, or if they feel self-conscious about the difference.

Parents, caregivers, and educators must prepare children for these moments and equip them with strategies for handling intrusive or insensitive questions. One approach is to role-play different scenarios with the child, offering them options for how they can respond. For example, a child might respond with something like, "I have a special story about how I was born, but it's personal, and I'm happy to share it when I feel ready." This response validates the child's story while also setting a boundary for personal privacy.

Another approach is to help the child feel comfortable with their story, regardless of what others may say. By emphasizing the positive aspects of their family structure—such as the love and support they receive from their parents—children are less likely to internalize negative comments or feel insecure about their origins. Teaching children how to respond with confidence can turn a potentially awkward situation into a learning opportunity for others.

When peers ask questions, it's also important to teach children how to educate others in a way that is both informative and non-confrontational. For example, the child might say, "Some people have different types of families, and I was lucky to have a family who loves me very much." This approach doesn't go into unnecessary detail but helps others understand that family structures can vary, and that all families are valuable and important.

Creating Safe Circles and Supportive Allies

To support donor-conceived children in their social environments, it's vital to create safe circles of friends, teachers, and community members who are empathetic, accepting, and informed. Peer relationships are critical during childhood and adolescence, and having a strong support system in place can make a significant difference in the child's emotional well-being.

Safe circles can be cultivated through open conversations and inclusive activities. For example, in schools, teachers can incorporate lessons about diverse family structures and encourage students to share their family stories. This could include discussing different ways families are made, including donor conception, adoption, and blended families. These conversations help normalize diversity and provide a safe space for children to discuss their family experiences without feeling singled out or misunderstood.

In addition to school environments, social circles of friends who are understanding and non-judgmental can create a supportive network for donor-conceived children. It's important for parents to help their child cultivate friendships where the focus is on shared interests, values, and mutual respect, rather than on differences in family structure. These friendships can offer emotional support and act as a buffer against insensitive comments or isolation.

Encouraging supportive allies is another important aspect of fostering a positive social environment. Allies are individuals who stand up for others and help create an inclusive atmosphere. This can include teachers, friends, extended family, or even classmates who understand and appreciate the unique challenges that donor-conceived children may face. Allies can advocate for the child in social settings, help address insensitive questions, and provide emotional support when needed.

Parents can also connect their child with other donor-conceived individuals, either through community groups, online forums, or local meet-ups. These connections help the child see that they are not alone in their experiences and offer opportunities to build friendships with others who share similar family dynamics.

Creating a supportive environment in both school and social settings is critical in helping donor-conceived children feel understood and accepted. The more positive interactions they have with their peers and mentors, the more confident they will feel in navigating their identity and their unique family story.

Conclusion

As donor-conceived children grow, the role of culture, community, and representation in shaping their sense of self cannot be overstated. The need for donor-conceived characters and stories in media, literature, and everyday conversations is essential in normalizing their experience and helping them see themselves as valid and important members of society. When donor-conceived children are able to see their family structure reflected in books, TV shows, and movies, they are more likely to develop a healthy sense of self and a strong feeling of belonging.

In social settings like school and with friends, navigating curiosity and insensitive questions requires preparation, confidence, and the support of safe circles and allies. By fostering inclusive environments and creating spaces for open conversations, parents, educators, and communities can help donor-conceived children thrive socially and emotionally.

Ultimately, creating a world where donor-conceived children feel seen, understood, and valued is about embracing diversity in all its forms and ensuring that every child has the opportunity to grow up with pride in their story, no matter how their family was made.

Chapter 10

Parent Identity and Emotional Processing

Introduction:

Parenthood is a transformative journey, one that redefines individuals and reshapes their identities. For parents of donor-conceived children, this journey can be marked by complex emotional landscapes, where grief, loss, and the relinquishment of biological ties intersect with profound love, acceptance, and the joy of parenthood. While the experience of becoming a parent through donor conception can be incredibly rewarding, it often requires emotional processing that is unique to this path. Parents may face grief over infertility or the loss of the dream of biological parenthood, and they may need to navigate their feelings about the biological origins of their child.

In this chapter, we will explore the emotional journey that parents of donor-conceived children experience as they reconcile their identities as parents and process the emotions tied to donor conception. In Section 1, we delve into the emotional stages that parents often go through, from grief to grace, as they process infertility, loss, and the letting go of biological connections. We will also explore how these emotions shape the family narrative. In Section 2, we will discuss how parents can build stronger bonds with their child through empathy, transparency, and emotional availability, while avoiding the pitfalls of overcompensation or silence. Understanding and processing these emotions is crucial for parents to navigate their journey with authenticity, fostering a strong and healthy family dynamic.

Section 1: From Grief to Grace

Processing Infertility, Loss, and Letting Go of Biology

For many parents, the path to donor conception begins with infertility or the realization that biological parenthood is not possible or may not be the path they had envisioned. Infertility can be an emotionally taxing journey, filled with cycles of hope and disappointment. It can lead to feelings of inadequacy, frustration, and grief. These emotions are valid and should be acknowledged, as they often shape the way parents approach the idea of donor conception.

Grief is one of the most common emotions parents face when dealing with infertility. It is the mourning of the loss of the dream of having a child through biological means, the loss of genetic continuity, and the loss of the family structure they had envisioned. For some parents, this grief can be profound, as it challenges deeply held assumptions about family, identity, and legacy. The experience of infertility often brings feelings of helplessness and disillusionment, particularly when various treatments fail or the cause of infertility remains unexplained. These feelings of loss can last long after the decision to pursue donor conception is made, and may linger as the parent grapples with what their family will look like and how they will relate to their child.

Letting go of the idea of biological parenthood and embracing donor conception requires emotional processing that can take time. Some parents might feel conflicted about whether they are "real" parents if they are not biologically related to their child. These emotions are valid and must be addressed to ensure a healthy adjustment to the new family structure. Letting go of biology can feel like an emotional surrender, but it also allows for a different kind of connection—one rooted in love and choice, rather than biology alone.

For many parents, this process requires reframing their understanding of parenthood. Biological parenthood often comes with societal and cultural assumptions about what it means to be a parent, but in the case of donor conception, the path to becoming a parent is based on intentionality, love, and commitment. Embracing donor conception means acknowledging that biological connections, while important, do not define the essence of parenting. The parent-child bond is shaped by caregiving, emotional presence, and the deep affection shared between parent and child.

In many ways, this shift from biology to intentionality can be empowering. Parents begin to realize that the love they offer their child is what defines them as parents. This realization can ease the grief of infertility and help parents move toward acceptance and grace in their journey. The emotional growth that comes with processing infertility and letting go of the idea of biological parenthood is a critical part of the family's narrative. It is an evolution from a place of loss to one of grace, where parents embrace the new identity of parenthood with a sense of purpose and joy.

Parents who process their grief fully and allow themselves the time to heal are better equipped to create a healthy, loving environment for their donor-conceived child. They can approach the parenting experience with greater emotional resilience and a sense of peace, knowing that their journey to parenthood was not defined by biology, but by the love they offer their child.

Understanding How Your Emotions Shape the Narrative

Parents' emotions around donor conception inevitably shape the family narrative. The way parents feel about their fertility journey, their relationship with the donor, and their emotional connection to their child will inform how they talk about their family and, ultimately, how the child understands their story.

When parents are able to process their emotions, they can create a family narrative that is rich in love, meaning, and understanding. A family story that acknowledges the grief of infertility and the joy of parenthood through donor conception will help children understand their origins in a healthy, balanced way. Children will grow up knowing that their family was created with love, thoughtfulness, and intention—regardless of the biological connection.

How parents communicate about their emotional processing also sets the tone for the child's understanding of their identity. If parents have not fully processed their own feelings of grief or loss, it may inadvertently affect how they talk about the donor, the family story, or their child's origins. Children are highly sensitive to the emotions of their parents and may pick up on subtle cues that could affect their sense of self-worth or identity. On the other hand, when parents are emotionally available, transparent, and grounded in their own narrative, they can provide a stable foundation for their child to develop their own understanding of who they are and where they come from.

Parents need to give themselves permission to express their emotions openly, while also offering their child the opportunity to process their feelings about donor conception in their own time. This creates an emotionally healthy family dynamic in which both the parents and the child feel supported, loved, and understood.

Section 2: Building Stronger Bonds

Empathy, Transparency, and Emotional Availability

Once parents have processed their own emotions surrounding donor conception, they are better able to be emotionally available to their child. Emotional availability means being present with the child—listening to their concerns, answering their questions, and providing reassurance when needed. Donor-conceived children often have questions about their biological origins, and it's important for parents to respond with empathy and understanding, rather than with defensiveness or discomfort.

Empathy is a crucial aspect of this emotional availability. Parents need to acknowledge the child's feelings and provide validation for their experiences, whether those feelings are of curiosity, confusion, or even frustration. It's normal for donor-conceived children to feel a sense of difference or wonder about their biological parent. By empathizing with these feelings and offering support, parents can help their child navigate the complex emotional landscape that comes with understanding their origins.

Transparency is equally important. As children grow older and begin to ask more questions about their donor, it's essential for parents to provide clear, age-appropriate answers that are truthful yet sensitive. Transparency doesn't mean providing all the details immediately; rather, it means offering information in a way that respects the child's emotional readiness. When parents are transparent, it builds trust and fosters an open, honest relationship in which the child feels safe to explore their questions and emotions.

Parents should also be open to discussing their own emotions regarding donor conception, when appropriate. Sharing feelings of gratitude, love, and intentionality helps the child understand that their family was created out of a deep, conscious choice. At the same time, parents should also acknowledge that, while they may not have been able to conceive biologically, their bond with the child is no less profound or meaningful.

However, parents should avoid the extremes of overcompensation or silence. Overcompensation can occur when parents attempt to make up for the absence of a biological connection by over-indulging or placing too much pressure on the child. This might manifest in excessive efforts to prove their love or provide an "ideal" family experience. While love and care are essential, trying too hard to make everything perfect can create unnecessary pressure on both the child and the parent.

On the other hand, silence—whether it's about donor conception, infertility, or emotions surrounding parenthood—can be just as damaging. Avoiding the topic entirely may lead to feelings of isolation or confusion for the child. Silence may also prevent the child from feeling like they have permission to explore their feelings about donor conception. It's essential for parents to strike a balance between being emotionally available and being honest about their journey, without overwhelming the child with too much information or too many expectations.

Avoiding Overcompensation or Silence

Navigating the balance between overcompensation and silence requires emotional awareness and self-reflection. Parents should examine their motivations and feelings when interacting with their child about donor conception. Overcompensation often comes from a place of guilt or anxiety over the lack of biological ties, while silence may stem from discomfort or fear of making the child feel "different."

In these moments, it's important to recognize that the child's sense of identity and family can remain secure without feeling pressure or secrecy. A healthy family narrative is one in which the child feels loved, valued, and understood, without the need to prove that their family is any "better" or "worse" than others. Avoiding extremes means providing a steady, loving foundation where the child is encouraged to ask questions and express emotions while knowing that their place in the family is unwavering.

Parents can build stronger bonds with their child by fostering an emotionally supportive environment, being transparent about their own feelings, and responding with empathy and love to the child's emotional needs. Creating a family dynamic that is open, nurturing, and accepting will help donor-conceived children feel confident in their identity, secure in their place within the family, and empowered to explore their biological origins on their terms.

Conclusion

The emotional journey of becoming a parent through donor conception is a multifaceted process that involves navigating grief, loss, and ultimately, acceptance and grace. Parents must process their own emotions about infertility and the lack of biological connection in order to build a strong, emotionally healthy relationship with their donor-conceived child. By fostering empathy, transparency, and emotional availability, parents can create a family dynamic that allows the child to develop a secure and integrated sense of identity. At the same time, parents must be mindful of avoiding overcompensation or silence, ensuring that their approach is balanced and grounded in love. By embracing the emotional complexities of their journey and creating a supportive environment, parents of donor-conceived children can help nurture strong, resilient bonds that will endure as the child grows and explores their own identity.

Chapter 11

Building the Child's Narrative with Strength

Introduction:

Parenting is a journey of guiding children through their emotional and psychological development, helping them form their own sense of identity and belonging. For parents of donor-conceived children, this journey includes not only supporting their child's growth but also co-creating their narrative—one that acknowledges the child's origins, celebrates their unique family story, and fosters strength and resilience. How children understand and integrate their origins into their sense of self is crucial in shaping their emotional health and self-confidence.

This chapter explores how parents can help donor-conceived children build a strong narrative about their origins. Section 1 focuses on the power of co-creating the child's story with them, using storytelling to build resilience and a sense of ownership over their identity. Section 2 shifts the focus to truth as a tool for confidence, emphasizing the importance of authenticity over secrecy. By fostering an open, honest, and positive family narrative, parents can help their children respond with pride and embrace their uniqueness.

Section 1: Co-Creating Their Story

Helping Children "Own" Their Origins

A child's sense of self is deeply influenced by the stories they hear about their beginnings—stories of where they come from, who their family members are, and the unique journey that brought them into the world. For donor-conceived children, their family story is often different from the traditional narratives they encounter in their peer groups, which may emphasize biological parent-child relationships. This makes it even more crucial for parents to **co-create** their child's story with them, fostering an active sense of ownership and pride in their origins.

One of the most important things parents can do is to start early in the child's life by introducing the concept of donor conception in a positive and affirming way. This could include simple phrases that frame the story in a positive light, such as, "You were made with the help of a very special person who wanted to help bring you into the world." These early conversations lay the groundwork for a family narrative that emphasizes love, intention, and choice, rather than biological connection alone.

As children grow older, it's essential for parents to include them in the narrative development. This doesn't mean overwhelming the child with information but rather helping them gradually build a story that resonates with them. This can be done by discussing the child's origins as part of their larger life story, highlighting the love and care that went into their conception, and showing how their family is special in its own right. When children feel included in the creation of their story, they are more likely to internalize it as a source of strength and confidence.

For instance, a parent might say, "Your donor played an important role in helping us create our family, but you are our child. You are part of us, and we love you deeply. We wanted you so much, and we are grateful every day for you." This statement not only provides a clear sense of the child's place within the family but also reinforces that their worth is not dependent on genetics but on the love and intentionality of the family they are a part of.

Ownership of the narrative also involves giving children the space to ask questions about their origins as they grow. As children become more aware of the differences in family structures, they may want to explore their own story further. By being open and receptive to these questions, parents show that the child's identity is fluid and adaptable—something that can evolve and grow with them. When children are allowed to actively engage with their narrative, they are empowered to make sense of their story in a way that fosters pride and confidence.

This process of co-creating the child's story also helps the family as a whole create a unified narrative. The family narrative doesn't just belong to the parents or to the child—it belongs to everyone who plays a part in the family dynamic. When the family shares a cohesive story, it strengthens the emotional bonds between parents and children and helps the child feel like a valued member of the family, regardless of their biological origins.

Using Storytelling to Build Resilience

Storytelling is a powerful tool for resilience-building. For children, particularly those who may feel different or experience moments of uncertainty about their origins, hearing a strong and positive narrative can help them develop emotional strength and a sense of identity. In this context, storytelling is not just about telling a family history—it's about framing that history in a way that fosters empowerment, pride, and a healthy sense of self.

For donor-conceived children, storytelling can provide a way to normalize their experience and help them feel that their family story is just as valuable and meaningful as any other. This is particularly important during times of emotional vulnerability, such as adolescence, when questions about identity and belonging are especially prominent.

A family narrative that highlights themes of choice, love, and connection rather than biological determinism can be a powerful antidote to feelings of inadequacy or confusion. For example, sharing stories about how the child's parents made a thoughtful, loving choice to bring them into the world through donor conception—rather than through the chance of biological circumstances—can foster a sense of pride and gratitude. Parents can tell the child how excited they were when they found out they were expecting, how much they wanted a child, and how their decision to pursue donor conception was an intentional act of love.

This storytelling also helps the child develop emotional resilience when faced with challenges or questions from peers. The child who has been told their story in a positive, empowering way is more likely to respond to questions with confidence, knowing that their family story is unique and valuable. Rather than feeling defensive or self-conscious, the child learns to take pride in their origins and respond to curiosity with a sense of self-assuredness.

In addition to empowering children to own their narrative, storytelling can help them understand the bigger picture of their identity. They come to understand that their family is a diverse, multifaceted entity, and their place within it is special and irreplaceable. By integrating storytelling into the family's daily life, parents ensure that their child's sense of self grows from a place of strength, resilience, and pride in their story.

Section 2: Truth as a Tool for Confidence

Authenticity Over Secrecy

For many parents, there may be a temptation to conceal certain details about their child's origins, especially when it comes to donor conception. This may stem from a fear of causing confusion, embarrassment, or unwanted attention. However, authenticity is the key to building a strong, resilient identity for the child. The more parents embrace honesty and transparency in their approach to explaining the child's origins, the stronger and more confident the child will become.

Secrecy around donor conception can lead to feelings of shame, alienation, and confusion. Children who are not told the truth about their origins may eventually sense that there is something hidden, and this can foster mistrust or insecurity. Worse still, if a child finds out the truth about their origins later in life, they may feel betrayed by their parents for keeping the information from them. This breach of trust can damage the parent-child relationship and may lead to emotional struggles during adolescence or adulthood.

In contrast, authenticity encourages a sense of self-worth and security. When children are raised in an environment where honesty is prioritized, they learn that their story—no matter how unconventional—is valid. This understanding is essential for building a sense of pride in who they are. By speaking openly about the donor's role and the family's journey, parents help their child internalize the idea that there is nothing shameful or wrong about their conception. It is simply one way of building a family, and it's a family full of love, care, and intentionality.

Honesty is also an important tool in helping the child process their emotions. When the truth is provided in a loving, age-appropriate way, the child can develop a deeper understanding of their feelings toward their donor and their family. For example, if a child feels sadness or confusion about not knowing their donor, parents can validate those feelings and offer reassurance. "It's okay to feel curious or unsure about your donor. Your feelings are valid, and I'm here to help you understand more about where you came from." This approach builds emotional security by showing the child that their feelings are important, and that they are not alone in their journey of self-discovery.

Helping Your Child Respond with Pride

As children grow older and begin to understand their donor conception more fully, they may face questions from peers, teachers, or even family members. How the child responds to these questions can be influenced by the narrative they've internalized. If they have been taught to view their story as special, meaningful, and worthy of pride, they are more likely to respond with confidence and self-assurance.

One way to help a child respond with pride is to frame their donor conception as part of their unique family story—one that is built on love and choice, rather than biology alone. Parents can empower their child by practicing responses to questions that reflect their confidence in their story. For instance, if a peer asks, "Who's your real dad?" the child can confidently respond, "I have a dad who loves me and took care of me. I was born with the help of a special donor who helped us become a family."

This type of response is not defensive but affirming. It allows the child to acknowledge their biological origins without feeling ashamed or uncomfortable. It also teaches others that there is nothing unusual or wrong about donor conception, reinforcing the idea that all families are valid, regardless of how they are formed.

Moreover, teaching the child to speak about their donor with respect and appreciation is crucial. If the donor is part of the child's narrative, they can be acknowledged in a way that reflects the importance of their role without idealizing or demonizing them. "My donor helped me be born, and I'm grateful for that. But my real family is the one that loves and cares for me every day."

This narrative helps the child embrace their story with pride and confidence. It also sets the stage for future conversations where the child can explore their feelings about their donor in an open, honest, and empowered way.

Conclusion

Building a strong, positive narrative around a donor-conceived child's origins is one of the most powerful ways parents can support their child's emotional development and self-confidence. By co-creating their story, parents help children feel ownership over their identity and develop a sense of pride in their uniqueness. Through storytelling, they can frame their family narrative in a way that emphasizes love, intention, and connection, fostering resilience in the face of any challenges. Authenticity and transparency are crucial tools for helping the child respond with confidence and pride, allowing them to navigate the world with a strong sense of self and a deep connection to their family story. By embracing honesty, love, and respect, parents can ensure that their donor-conceived child grows up feeling secure, valued, and proud of who they are.

Chapter 12
Voices of Donor-Conceived Adults

Introduction:

The journey of growing up as a donor-conceived child is unique, and the emotional complexities of this experience continue to evolve as children grow into adults. While much of the focus in the donor-conception community is on the parents and their role in helping their children navigate their origins, it is equally important to hear from the donor-conceived individuals themselves. Their stories offer valuable insights into the long-term impact of donor conception on identity, relationships, and emotional well-being. By understanding the lived experiences of donor-conceived adults, we can improve how we support children today and build a stronger, more informed framework for future generations.

This chapter is dedicated to the voices of donor-conceived adults, shedding light on their real experiences, struggles, and triumphs. In Section 1, we will explore their lived experiences, moving from confusion and uncertainty in their youth to greater clarity and acceptance in adulthood. We will also explore what these adults wish their parents had done differently in their upbringing, offering crucial lessons for those raising donor-conceived children today. In Section 2, we will dive into the insights, advice, and advocacy of donor-conceived adults, who are using their voices to support future generations and call for systemic changes that better serve the needs of donor-conceived individuals. These perspectives are instrumental in shaping how we move forward as a community, ensuring that donor-conceived individuals are heard, valued, and supported in all aspects of their lives.

Section 1: Lived Experiences

From Confusion to Clarity: Real Stories

The stories of donor-conceived adults are varied, but they share common threads of emotional growth, self-discovery, and a search for identity. For many donor-conceived individuals, the journey from confusion to clarity is a gradual process that evolves over time, shaped by their upbringing, their family dynamics, and their personal experiences with learning about their origins.

For some donor-conceived adults, the early years of life were marked by a lack of awareness or understanding of their donor origins. As children, they may have simply accepted the family narrative presented to them, trusting their parents and feeling loved and cared for. However, as they entered adolescence, the desire to understand their biological roots began to surface, often accompanied by confusion or a sense of difference.

"I always knew I was donor-conceived, but I didn't really understand what that meant until I was older," says Sarah, a donor-conceived adult. "I think it was when I hit my teenage years that it started to matter more. I looked around at my friends, and their families looked so similar. I didn't have that, and I didn't quite know how to make sense of it. It felt like something was missing, but I didn't know what it was."

For many adults, the process of learning about their origins is not a singular moment but rather a series of emotional milestones. The realization of being donor-conceived often unfolds gradually, influenced by the child's cognitive development, emotional maturity, and growing curiosity. While some children are told about their donor origins early in life, others may not learn the full story until adolescence or even adulthood.

Donor-conceived adults often express a range of emotions upon discovering or fully understanding their origins. Some feel a sense of relief or empowerment, finally understanding why they feel different or why they may not share certain traits with their social parents. Others feel anger, confusion, or betrayal if they were not told earlier in life or if they feel the narrative of their family was hidden from them. These reactions are entirely normal and reflect the complexity of processing a major aspect of one's identity.

"The hardest part for me was that I didn't know what to do with the information when I first found out," says Michael, another donor-conceived adult. "I didn't know how to feel about my donor. I had this sense of loss because I didn't know them, but at the same time, I felt like I was betraying my parents by being curious. It was a tough balance to figure out."

Over time, many donor-conceived adults come to terms with their origins and gain clarity about who they are. They learn to reconcile their biological and social connections, finding strength in their unique family stories. For many, this journey toward clarity involves accepting both their biological and social roots and realizing that their identity is shaped by more than just genetics.

Some donor-conceived individuals also undergo a reconnection process, seeking out biological relatives or discovering more about their donor's background. This can be a deeply emotional experience, one that brings a sense of connection and closure for some, while for others, it can raise new questions and create challenges in how they view their family dynamic. As adults, many donor-conceived individuals advocate for greater transparency and open access to information about their biological heritage, hoping to ensure that future generations of donor-conceived children have the opportunity to grow up with more clarity and understanding about their origins.

What They Wish Their Parents Had Done Differently

While many donor-conceived adults report having positive relationships with their social parents, they also reflect on what could have been done differently during their upbringing to help them better understand their origins and identity. For many, the key is early and ongoing communication about their donor conception, along with a family narrative that emphasizes acceptance, love, and honesty.

"I wish my parents had talked about the donor more openly and regularly," says Jessica, who learned about her donor conception at age 13. "It wasn't until I was a teenager that I really understood what being donor-conceived meant. By then, I had a lot of questions, but my parents weren't prepared to answer them. It felt like they were avoiding the subject, and that left me feeling like there was something to be ashamed of. I think if they'd been more open from the start, I wouldn't have felt so confused and alone."

Many donor-conceived adults express the importance of creating a family culture in which their origins are normalized and integrated into their identity from an early age. This includes openly discussing the donor's role in a positive, affirming way, without making it the focal point of the child's identity but rather one part of their broader family story. When parents overemphasize or underemphasize the donor's role, it can create emotional turmoil for the child as they grow older and develop a deeper understanding of family dynamics.

"I think it would have been helpful if my parents had been more transparent about their feelings," says Mark. "I could tell they were upset or conflicted about how I might feel about being donor-conceived. I think they were afraid I might feel rejected or unwanted. If they had just shared more about their own journey—what led them to make the decision to use a donor—it would have helped me understand that it was about love and choice, not about biology."

Parents of donor-conceived children should be mindful of not avoiding the subject or treating it as a "secret." In some cases, keeping the truth about a child's origins hidden can create unnecessary tension and confusion. Openness and transparency, paired with emotional support, can help children feel more secure in their identity and more confident in understanding their place in the world.

Section 2: Insights, Advice, and Advocacy

Speaking for Future Generations

As donor-conceived adults reflect on their own experiences, many are committed to speaking out and advocating for the rights and well-being of future generations. They are using their voices to ensure that the emotional needs of donor-conceived children are addressed and that their rights to information, transparency, and connection to their biological origins are recognized.

One of the most common pieces of advice from donor-conceived adults is the importance of early education and honest communication. They urge parents of donor-conceived children to normalize conversations about donor conception from an early age, creating a family environment where questions are welcomed and explored with respect and love.

"I think the biggest thing I would say to parents is to be open," says Emily, a donor-conceived adult. "You don't have to have all the answers, but being open to talking about it as part of their story will make a huge difference. Don't make it something to hide or be ashamed of. The earlier you talk about it, the better. It helps the child grow up with confidence in who they are and pride in their story."

Another key issue raised by donor-conceived adults is the need for greater access to genetic information. Many donor-conceived individuals express frustration over their inability to access detailed information about their donor or biological relatives, particularly if they were conceived using an anonymous donor. Advocacy for donor anonymity laws is central to the movement for greater transparency, as many donor-conceived adults believe that knowing about their biological origins is essential for both their physical and emotional well-being.

"Not having access to information about my donor has always felt like a void," says Alex, a donor-conceived adult. "I don't know if my donor is still alive, what health conditions run in my biological family, or even what my donor looks like. That's a lot to navigate emotionally. I think every donor-conceived person should have the right to know about their origins."

Changing Systems and Supporting Others

The experiences of donor-conceived adults are also driving systemic change within the donor conception industry. Many advocate for stricter regulations, better donor tracking, and clearer legal frameworks to protect the rights of donor-conceived children. Their goal is to ensure that future generations have access to the information they need to make informed decisions about their health, identity, and relationships.

One area of advocacy is around open donor systems, where donors are no longer anonymous, allowing donor-conceived individuals to have access to information about their biological parentage. Advocates argue that anonymity should not come at the cost of a child's right to know about their origins and that future generations should not have to navigate the emotional difficulties of growing up without answers to their basic questions.

"The system needs to change," says Olivia, another donor-conceived adult. "We're talking about people's identities, their health, and their rights. This is not something that should be treated as a business transaction or a secret. We deserve to know about our biological family. The more we talk about this, the more pressure we can put on the system to change."

In addition to systemic advocacy, many donor-conceived adults are also engaged in supporting others in their community. They participate in online forums, support groups, and advocacy organizations to offer advice, share their stories, and provide emotional support to donor-conceived individuals who may be struggling with their identity or family dynamics.

"Being a part of a community of people who understand what it's like to be donor-conceived has been so helpful for me," says Sarah. "It's a safe space where I can talk about my feelings without feeling judged or misunderstood. I think everyone who's donor-conceived should have that support, so they know they're not alone."

Conclusion

The voices of donor-conceived adults offer invaluable insights into the long-term emotional and psychological impact of donor conception. Their stories, shaped by a journey from confusion to clarity, provide important lessons for both parents and advocates. Through their advocacy, they are working to ensure that future generations of donor-conceived individuals have greater access to information, transparency, and emotional support.

Chapter 13

The Path Forward – Empowerment Over Explanation

Introduction:

Parenthood is a journey filled with love, growth, and the constant development of a unique family story. For parents of donor-conceived children, this path is deeply enriching but also requires a nuanced approach to help children form a strong, secure, and positive sense of self. Raising a donor-conceived child involves more than simply explaining where they came from—it requires fostering empowerment. Empowerment isn't about providing simple answers to complex questions about identity, but about nurturing a child's confidence, sense of belonging, and self-worth regardless of biological ties.

As society shifts towards more inclusive, open-minded views of family creation, it is imperative that we move beyond mere explanation and towards creating a family narrative that celebrates love, choice, and intentionality. This narrative will help children grow into secure, self-aware individuals who understand that their family is not defined by biology but by love, connection, and shared history.

In this chapter, we will explore how parents can foster an environment of empowerment and authenticity for their donor-conceived children. In Section 1, we will look at how to build a legacy of truth and love by raising children who are secure in their identities, self-aware, and connected to their family. We will also discuss how to shift from secrecy to celebration, and why this change in perspective is so important. In Section 2, we will examine the resources, support systems, and communities available to both parents and donor-conceived children, including books, therapists, networks, and organizations that help families navigate this journey. These resources are essential in helping families thrive, both emotionally and psychologically.

Section 1: Creating a Legacy of Truth and Love

Raising Secure, Self-Aware, and Connected Children

Raising secure, self-aware, and connected children begins with an environment that fosters emotional safety, trust, and unconditional love. For donor-conceived children, the emotional foundations of their identity are laid in the early years, where parents must strike a delicate balance between providing age-appropriate information about their origins and building a stable sense of self.

The first step in raising a secure child is establishing a relationship based on unconditional love. This love, while certainly not unique to donor-conceived children, becomes even more vital when biological ties are not present. When parents make clear that the love and care they provide are not conditional on genetics, the child learns to value themselves for who they are rather than where they came from. In many ways, love becomes the central theme of the child's narrative—the cornerstone of their identity. A child who grows up feeling loved and valued will be better equipped to handle the complexities of their origins, even as they become more aware of the biological aspects of their family story.

Equally important is fostering self-awareness in the child. This involves encouraging them to ask questions, explore their feelings, and develop a positive sense of who they are. In donor-conceived children, this sense of self-awareness may take a little longer to develop, especially when the child begins to understand that their family structure is different from that of their peers. However, self-awareness isn't just about accepting that they are donor-conceived—it's about helping them embrace the broader aspects of their identity, both biological and social.

Self-awareness also includes helping children recognize that they are part of a larger family narrative—one that transcends biology and is built on love, intentionality, and connection. Parents can instill this understanding by discussing the family's story from a very young age, emphasizing that while their family may be different, it is just as meaningful and important as any other. This foundation of truth helps children see themselves not as "different" but as a unique and integral part of their family.

Connection is the third essential element in raising a secure, self-aware, and emotionally healthy child. This involves fostering strong relationships within the family, with peers, and with the larger community. For donor-conceived children, connection can sometimes feel uncertain, especially if they are the only child in their peer group with a non-traditional family structure. As parents, it is crucial to model openness, acceptance, and inclusivity, showing the child that family is not just about biology, but about emotional bonds and shared experiences.

When children feel connected—both to their family and to a larger community of people who support them—they develop a more robust sense of self. This connection can be nurtured through family activities, open communication, and a sense of belonging in both their immediate family and the wider community. Whether it's through relationships with extended family, close friends, or participation in social and community groups, feeling connected is essential to fostering emotional security.

Shifting from Secrecy to Celebration

For many years, donor conception was often treated as a subject to be kept secret—a private matter to be disclosed only when necessary or when the child was older. This practice stemmed in part from a desire to protect the child, as well as concerns about how others might perceive the family. However, secrecy creates an emotional burden for children, who may sense that there is something about their origins that is not to be talked about openly. As a result, the absence of open discussion can lead to confusion, anxiety, and a sense of shame.

The key to moving forward with empowerment is to shift from secrecy to celebration—to create an environment where donor conception is embraced as part of the family's story, rather than something to hide or downplay. This shift allows donor-conceived children to grow up with a healthy understanding of their origins and feel secure in their identity. It also encourages them to approach their story with pride, knowing that their family was formed with love, intention, and care.

One of the most powerful ways to celebrate donor conception is through language. The language parents use when talking about their child's origins is crucial. Instead of speaking about donor conception as a "complicated" or "difficult" subject, parents should frame it as a beautiful, intentional process that led to the creation of a loving family. This positive language helps the child develop a sense of pride in their origins rather than feeling that they are somehow "less than" or "different" from other children.

For example, instead of saying, "We couldn't have children naturally, so we had to go to a donor," parents might say, "We really wanted you, and so we made the loving decision to bring you into the world with the help of a very special person. You are a part of our family because we chose you, and that makes you incredibly important to us." This kind of language reinforces the idea that the child is loved, chosen, and valued, and that their family is just as meaningful as any other.

Celebrating donor conception also involves including the child in the family story from a young age. Parents can talk openly about the donor's role and explain how their family was formed, always emphasizing that love, not biology, is the foundation of family. The child's sense of pride in their family story will grow as they understand that their family, though different, is just as full of love and connection as any other.

Honoring the Donor's Role

Another important aspect of celebration is honoring the donor's role. The donor helped create the child's life, and while they may not be part of the child's daily life, their contribution is meaningful. Parents can celebrate the donor's role in ways that feel appropriate for the family's situation. If the donor is known, parents can talk about the donor's generosity and the special role they played. If the donor is anonymous, parents can still celebrate the fact that their family was intentionally created, even if the donor's identity is not part of the equation.

Honoring the donor's role does not mean idolizing them or placing them above the child's social parents. Instead, it's about recognizing the donor's contribution as part of the larger family story. This helps the child understand that their family story is rich and multifaceted, and it can lead to feelings of gratitude and appreciation for the many ways their family was made.

Section 2: Resources, Support, and Community

Books, Therapists, Networks, and Online Spaces

Support and resources are essential for families navigating the complexities of donor conception. Books designed for both children and parents can offer guidance, provide affirming narratives, and open the door for conversations about identity and origins. Children's books about donor conception, like *"The Family Book"* by Todd Parr or *"My Family is Special"* by David Hill, are great tools for opening up the subject in a simple, accessible way. These books celebrate the diversity of family structures and emphasize that love is the foundation of any family, regardless of how it was formed.

For parents, there are numerous resources available that offer practical advice, emotional support, and insights into the unique challenges of raising a donor-conceived child. Books like *"The Gift of Life"* by Kate Bourne and *"Donor-Conceived Children: Identity and the Right to Know"* by Fiona Kelly are valuable resources for learning more about the emotional, legal, and social aspects of donor conception.

Therapists and counselors specializing in reproductive health, identity, and family dynamics can also provide essential support. Therapy can be particularly helpful when the family faces challenges related to identity, secrecy, or the child's emotional struggles with their origins. A therapist can offer a safe space for both parents and children to explore their feelings, resolve conflicts, and develop coping strategies for navigating their unique family dynamics.

Online networks and support groups provide a sense of community for donor-conceived families. Websites like the Donor Sibling Registry and forums such as DonorConception.com offer opportunities for donor-conceived individuals and their families to connect with others who share similar experiences. These online spaces offer emotional support, a platform for exchanging advice, and a way to connect with others who may have similar questions or concerns about donor conception.

Social media groups and communities, such as Facebook groups dedicated to donor-conceived families, also offer a space for parents and children to share their stories, resources, and experiences. These platforms foster a sense of belonging and provide a way for individuals to find support and solidarity in their experiences.

Organizations Supporting Donor-Conceived Families

In addition to books and online communities, there are several organizations that advocate for the rights and well-being of donor-conceived individuals. Organizations like the Donor Conception Network (DCN) in the UK and The American Society for Reproductive Medicine (ASRM) in the U.S. provide resources, guidance, and support for families navigating the world of donor conception.

These organizations work to raise awareness about the emotional and psychological needs of donor-conceived individuals, advocate for openness and transparency in the donor conception process, and offer practical advice for families. They also serve as advocacy groups, pushing for policies that support donor-conceived individuals' rights to access information about their biological origins and advocating for changes in the donor conception industry to ensure better practices and ethical standards.

Another important organization is The Open Birth Records Coalition, which advocates for the rights of donor-conceived individuals to have access to the information about their biological parents. This movement seeks to ensure that donor-conceived individuals have the same rights to information as adopted children, helping to shift societal and legal norms towards greater transparency in the donor conception process.

These organizations not only provide support for families but also help to create a collective voice for donor-conceived individuals. Their advocacy work is pushing for systemic changes that will benefit future generations of donor-conceived children, ensuring they grow up in a world where transparency, support, and ethical practices are the norm.

Conclusion

The path forward for donor-conceived families is one of empowerment, rooted in truth, love, and celebration. By raising secure, self-aware, and connected children, parents can help their children develop a strong sense of identity that embraces both their biological and social roots. Moving from secrecy to celebration allows families to create a legacy that is built on openness, acceptance, and pride in their unique story.

Moreover, the resources, support systems, and communities available to families play a critical role in ensuring the emotional well-being of both parents and children. From books and therapy to online networks and advocacy organizations, these tools provide the guidance, solidarity, and practical advice that families need to navigate the challenges of donor conception.

As we look forward, the goal should be to create a world where donor-conceived children are raised with pride in their family story, where transparency and support are the foundation, and where their emotional needs are met with understanding, love, and respect. This is the path forward—one of empowerment, authenticity, and a deep, unshakable sense of belonging.

Epilogue

The journey of supporting donor-conceived children in forming strong, integrated identities is a deeply transformative process, not only for the children themselves but for the families, educators, and clinicians who guide them along the way. Throughout this book, we've explored the essential elements that contribute to the healthy identity development of donor-conceived children, from the foundational aspects of their identity to the ways in which they navigate their unique family stories.

In Chapter 1, we began by examining the intricate relationship between genes, environment, and storytelling in shaping who we are. We recognized that the traditional debate of nature versus nurture has evolved, and now we understand that for donor-conceived children, their identities are shaped by both biological connections and the love and care provided by their social parents. Their story matters, not just because of the biological factors but because of the intentionality and emotional depth of the family that raises them.

As we moved through the subsequent chapters, we explored the broader landscape of donor conception, from its historical roots to the current global conversation around anonymous and open donation. These discussions highlighted the shifting dynamics in reproductive technologies, laws, and cultural perceptions, underscoring the importance of transparent communication about biological origins for future generations.

Chapters 3 and 4 delved into the psychological effects of knowing or not knowing about one's biological origins. These sections illuminated the emotional complexities donor-conceived children face, from confusion and curiosity to the pivotal moments of truth. The way parents approach these conversations, with empathy and careful consideration of the child's developmental stage, plays a critical role in fostering resilience and emotional well-being.

We then explored the unique dynamics within the family unit in Chapter 7, emphasizing the power of love over biology in forming strong, secure bonds. In particular, the role of social parents in building attachment, answering difficult questions, and navigating sibling relationships is vital in creating an environment where children feel emotionally secure and valued, no matter their biological background.

In Chapter 8, we reflected on the emotional milestones throughout childhood and adolescence, acknowledging that the process of discovering one's identity involves significant shifts and emotional growth. From toddlers beginning to notice differences to teens searching for wholeness, each stage of development is crucial in helping children understand their origins, cope with any challenges, and build emotional resilience.

Chapters 9 and 10 focused on the importance of representation in the world around donor-conceived children. Normalizing their experiences in media, books, and social settings helps them feel seen and validated. This chapter also reinforced the need for parents to process their own emotions surrounding donor conception, ensuring that they can support their child's emotional needs with empathy, transparency, and openness.

By the time we reached Chapter 11, we learned that storytelling is a powerful tool in shaping the child's narrative, helping them take ownership of their story with pride and confidence. With the right guidance, donor-conceived children can come to see their origins not as a source of confusion or shame but as part of a rich, meaningful family story built on love and intention.

In Chapter 12, we heard the voices of donor-conceived adults, whose lived experiences offer valuable lessons for both parents and professionals. Their reflections and advocacy highlight the ongoing need for systemic changes, transparency, and greater access to information for donor-conceived individuals.

Finally, in Chapter 13, we focused on the path forward. Empowerment over explanation is the ultimate goal—creating a legacy where children feel secure in their identity, confident in their origins, and celebrated for who they are. Shifting from secrecy to celebration is the key to fostering environments where donor-conceived children can thrive emotionally and psychologically. By providing access to resources, support, and community, we ensure that donor-conceived children, their families, and advocates have the tools they need to navigate this journey with pride and confidence.

As we move forward, the focus must be on nurturing these children with love, honesty, and emotional support, while ensuring that families and communities have access to the resources and information necessary to support their growth. The future of donor-conceived children depends not on how we explain their origins, but on how we empower them to embrace their identities with pride, strength, and resilience.

www.ingramcontent.com/pod-product-compliance
Lightning Source LLC
Chambersburg PA
CBHW071521120626

46550CB00006B/2309